CHI KUNG
for
RADIANT SKIN

"Master Chia and Anna Margolina, Ph.D., have done an excellent job of explaining the skin as our third lung as well as describing how to clean and maintain the skin from the inside out with Taoist Chi Kung and meditations."

WILLIAM. U. WEI,
SENIOR INSTRUCTOR OF THE UNIVERSAL TAO
AND COAUTHOR OF *THE TAO OF IMMORTALITY*
AND *LIVING IN THE TAO*

Chi Kung
for
Radiant Skin

Taoist Secrets for
Inner and Outer Beauty

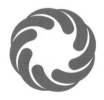

Mantak Chia
and
Anna Margolina, Ph.D.

Destiny Books
Rochester, Vermont

Destiny Books
One Park Street
Rochester, Vermont 05767
www.DestinyBooks.com

Destiny Books is a division of Inner Traditions International

Originally published in Thailand in 2022 by Universal Healing Tao Publications under the title *Beauty Chi Kung: Taoist Secrets of Radiant Skin*

Cataloging-in-Publication Data for this title is available from the Library of Congress

ISBN 978-1-64411-757-6 (print)
ISBN 978-1-64411-758-3 (ebook)

Printed and bound in India at Replika Press Pvt. Ltd.

10 9 8 7 6 5 4 3 2 1

Text design by Priscilla Baker and layout by K. Manseau
This book was typeset in Garamond Premier Pro with Present Sho and Futura used as display typefaces

To send correspondence to the authors of this book, mail a first-class letter to the authors c/o Inner Traditions • Bear & Company, One Park Street, Rochester, VT 05767, and we will forward the communication.

Scan the QR code and save 25% at InnerTraditions.com. Browse over 2,000 titles on spirituality, the occult, ancient mysteries, new science, holistic health, and natural medicine.

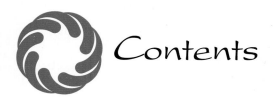

Contents

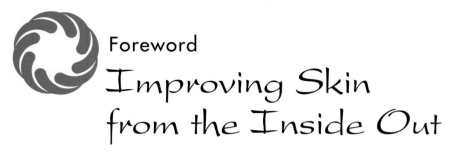

Foreword

Improving Skin from the Inside Out

Jutta Kellenberger-Reichert

This book is for anyone interested in understanding and improving the quality of their skin. It features a Western scientific perspective alongside time-tested Taoist wisdom. Master Mantak Chia is the world's leading authority on Taoist energy practices; Anna Margolina, Ph.D., has studied the mind, body, and skin, both as a scientist and in relation to her background in Taoist energy practices, as a dedicated practitioner and certified Universal Healing Tao instructor with many years of experience.

The energy practices described in this book, which are based on first transforming and balancing the emotions inside our own physical body, have been practiced by Taoist masters for thousands of years. Master Mantak Chia, who has studied both traditional Taoist wisdom and modern Western medicine, dedicated decades to developing his science-based approach to Taoist inner alchemy teachings, resulting in a discipline that perfectly responds to the needs of our times. When practiced, the methods result in the body becoming less energetically dense, allowing for the absorption of more energy from nature and the universe for self-healing.

Today many people in the Western world already understand that consumerism does not create more happiness and is destructive to the body, mind, and planet. As people live longer, they are redefining aging and looking for new ways to transform and improve their lives and bodies. The premise of this book is that one's health is reflected in the quality of their skin. Just from observing a person's skin it is possible to see much deeper aspects of the person's physical health, emotional state, and energy level. In many cases the reason why the skin has lost its tone and become flabby, tense, or dry is not biological skin aging, but inner imbalance. Instead of applying different creams, lotions, or other topical remedies for different skin problems, Taoist masters throughout the ages have taught students to work on such problems from the inside out, practicing specific meditation practices for energy transformation and organ detox. The important takeaway from these inner alchemy practices is that an overall improvement of one's health and emotions will rejuvenate the skin, which shows in improved elasticity and radiance.

In this book, Master Mantak Chia and Anna Margolina address many of the most important elements of beautiful skin, such as the important role of nutrition, the role the emotions play in skin beauty, the cultivation of sexual energy to enhance beauty, and other aspects that impact the skin's vibrancy, health, and aesthetics.

I am truly excited about this book because it helped me solve a mystery that has puzzled me over the years. I have very fair, thin skin that never tans, and which, as I now know, requires protection from the sun, otherwise it ages very quickly. When I was in my twenties I started windsurfing. Since I didn't know much about the damaging effects of the sun, I surfed without sun protection and in bright sunlight, so I suffered frequent sunburns. Now that I am much older my skin *should* be severely damaged—but instead it is healthy and vibrant as a result of practicing the Universal Healing Tao for over thirty years!

In teaching this sublime ancient practice over the last twenty-two years I have had many students tell me wonderful stories about healing themselves using the methods of the Taoist masters. I have met people who have healed their relationships, addictions, and even such serious health conditions as cancer. Of course, Chi Kung is not a substitute for qualified medical care; however it can help make any treatment more effective by restoring the body's natural, innate ability to heal itself.

When we cultivate self-love, eat fresh and healthy food, chew well before swallowing, and practice internal Chi Kung practices to move energy in the body, we restore balance and flow in the body to bring forth vitality.

Today we are privileged to be able to access the vast knowledge of Taoist energy mastery and understand it through the lens of Western science and anatomy. Once secret knowledge, available to only a few, today these Taoist practices can be a part of your daily lifestyle. I truly believe that one's inner beauty shines through the skin and creates true and timeless outer beauty. This book is a practical guide to achieving that goal.

JUTTA KELLENBERGER-REICHERT is an International Universal Healing Tao teacher dedicated to helping people of all ages become strong, healthy, spiritual beings through Taoist energy practices. She has been a student of Master Chia since 1987 and a senior instructor of Taoist teachings since 2001. She lives in Barcelona, Spain, and travels around the world to teach workshops and connect with students. The author of *How to Develop Inner Beauty and Outer Radiance* (available in several languages), some of her course offerings are available online at **juttakellenberger.com**.

Acknowledgments

The authors and Universal Healing Tao Publications staff involved in the preparation and production of *Chi Kung for Radiant Skin: Taoist Secrets for Inner and Outer Beauty* extend our gratitude to the many generations of Taoist masters who have passed on their special knowledge, in the form of an unbroken oral transmission, over thousands of years. In particular we thank Taoist Master Yi Eng, known as the One Cloud Hermit, for his openness in transmitting the most sacred formulas of Taoist Inner Alchemy to Master Chia.

We offer eternal gratitude and love to our parents, who gave us life, and our teachers for their many gifts to us. Remembering them brings joy and satisfaction to our ongoing efforts in presenting the Universal Healing Tao system. As always, their contribution has been crucial in presenting the concepts and techniques of the Universal Healing Tao. We also wish to thank the thousands of unknown men and women of the Chinese healing arts who developed many of the methods and ideas presented in this book.

We send our special thanks to the many illustrators who contributed illustrations to this book, and we thank the many contributors who have been essential in bringing this book into final form: the editorial and production staff at Inner Traditions, for their efforts to clarify the text and produce a handsome new edition of the book, and Margaret Jones, for her line edit.

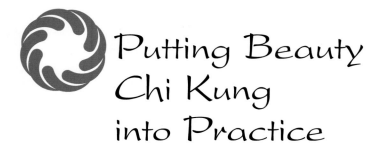

Putting Beauty Chi Kung into Practice

The information presented in this book is based on the authors' personal experience and knowledge. Many of the practices described here have been used successfully for thousands of years by Taoists trained by means of oral instruction, a teaching tradition that has been passed down through a long lineage of masters. Readers should not undertake these practices without receiving personal transmission and training from a certified instructor of the Universal Healing Tao, since certain of these practices, if done improperly, may cause injury or result in health problems. This book is intended to supplement individual training by the Universal Healing Tao and to serve as a reference guide for these practices. Anyone who undertakes these practices on the basis of this book alone does so entirely at his or her own risk.

The meditations, practices, and techniques described in this book are not intended to be used as an alternative to or substitute for professional medical treatment and care. If any readers are suffering from illnesses based on physical, mental, or emotional disorders, an appropriate professional health care practitioner or therapist should be consulted. Such problems should be corrected before you start Universal Healing Tao training.

Neither the Universal Healing Tao nor its staff and instructors are responsible for the consequences of any practice or misuse of the information contained in this book. If the reader undertakes any exercise without strictly following the instructions, notes, and warnings, the responsibility lies solely with the reader.

This book does not attempt to give any medical diagnosis, treatment, prescription, or remedial recommendation in relation to any human disease, ailment, suffering, or physical condition whatsoever.

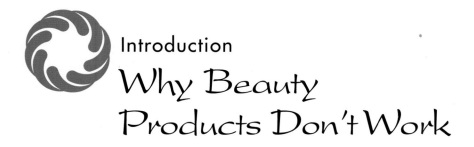

Introduction
Why Beauty Products Don't Work

Each year, approximately 49.2 billion dollars are generated in the United States by cosmetics sales, and on average Americans spend between $244 and $313 every month on cosmetics.[1] Department stores and cosmetic shops, drugstores, and the pages of women's magazines are full of alluring cosmetic products promising a youthful glow, smooth and radiant skin, and a flawless complexion. Many women cannot imagine life without their skin-care products and makeup. Whether they're used to conceal wrinkles, make the lips appear fuller and more seductive, create the illusion of bigger and more beautiful eyes, hide dark circles under the eyes, or conceal other tell-tale signs of aging, skin-care products are there to help us. Unfortunately, the older we get, the more difficult it is to conceal the signs of aging in the skin. Despite all the technological advances and methods of skin rejuvenation, many women and men remain deeply dissatisfied with the quality of their skin as they get older.* No matter what cosmetic product and no matter what cosmetic procedures we choose, achieving beautiful, radiant, vital-looking skin becomes increasingly difficult as we age.

---

*A December 14, 2022 article that appeared in *Cosmetics and Toiletries* reported that in a sampling of one thousand Americans it was found that regardless of spending habits, 67 percent of survey respondents worried about their appearance and 58 percent struggle with self-confidence. Weight, skin quality, and smile/teeth top the list of attributes American adults are self-conscious about. See "How Much Do Americans Spend on Their Looks Each Year?"

Beautiful skin is more than just an attractive façade for the human body. It is an integral part of one's personal expression, as it reflects the emotions and conditions of the body's organs. Healthy, resilient, well-nourished skin creates a sense of personal comfort and confidence. The reason why skin products and procedures have become as popular as they are is because good-looking, youthful, healthy, smooth skin has become a status symbol. A person with beautiful skin is often perceived as being more successful, wealthy, balanced, and even virtuous compared to a person with an uneven complexion, wrinkles, inflamed lesions, and coarse, rough skin.

For example, people who have the skin condition rosacea, which causes one's nose and cheeks to become red and inflamed, are often perceived as having a secret drinking habit or some other hidden vice—a judgment that can affect one's social acceptance and even employment. Skin is impossible to hide, and even though skin is an organ, it is also our outer shell, that which we present to the world. Healthy skin is an essential part of a professional, well-groomed appearance. No matter what people wear and no matter what qualifications they may have, it is ingrained in our human neurology to instantly notice a person's skin and its qualities. That's why many business professionals hire expensive photographers to ensure their headshot presents their best image to the outside world.

However if the face that appears on a business card or beautifully designed marketing brochure does not match the face people see in person, it creates a disconnect. It's not enough to look twenty years younger in promotional material, because there is no way anybody can hide their real skin from inquisitive eyes. No amount of makeup can mask unhealthy, lifeless skin or a bitter and displeased facial expression. Works of literature and glamour photographs on the pages of women's magazines acclaim the magical powers of youthful, soft, silky, smooth, delicate, flawless skin. To achieve the impossible perfection of eternal youth, many women and an increasing number of men are willing to invest money, time, and energy to try one "revolutionary" and "advanced" skin remedy after another, and many subject their skin to expensive, painful, invasive, risky surgical procedures.

Perhaps the desire to have beautiful, younger-looking skin may seem like vanity. However when skin rejuvenation is approached from a holistic perspective it can become the driving force for a healthier and more mindful lifestyle. What's more, the same practices that support beauty will also increase the body's resilience to viruses, age-related illnesses, and everyday stresses. Beauty and health are not separate; they support and feed each other. In a 2021 study it was discovered that elderly women who used skin-care products and makeup were less prone to falling down and had a lower risk of bone fractures.[2] Considering that for elderly people injuries resulting from falls can have dire consequences, this is a significant benefit. One reason simply *feeling* beautiful correlates with a much lower risk of falls is because such feelings generate a more balanced posture, inspired by greater self-confidence. Another is that people who feel more confident in their bodies go out more and connect more with other people. This leads to more natural physical movements such as walking, jogging, and even dancing. Feeling beautiful increases one's confidence and joy, which increases the production of endorphins, the "happy hormones." This makes

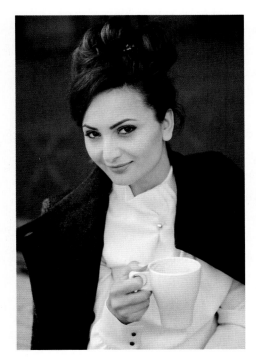

Figure I.1. Beautiful skin increases one's self-confidence and joy.

people want to connect with other people and thus prevents loneliness, which is proven to have many negative health consequences.[3] A person who feels beautiful and confident displays a welcoming, radiant energy that attracts people's attention and makes others more likely to approach them and start a conversation, which may lead to a beneficial business collaboration, friendship, or a more intimate soulmate connection.

The effects of aging on the skin is one of the main drivers behind why people buy skin-care products and undergo various procedures, some of them invasive. There are two main types of skin aging. One is genetically predetermined, or intrinsic skin aging; the other is aging caused by environmental and lifestyle factors, such as ultraviolet (UV) radiation and air pollution. Today, scientists know that not only UVB (290–320 nanometers, abbreviated *nm*) and UVA (320–400 nm) portions of solar radiation, but also visible[4] and infrared light[5] can cause skin damage and aging.[6] In industrially developed countries, air pollution, which includes smog and ozone and other toxic particles, has become one of the leading causes of premature skin aging.[7]

In 2020–21, during the COVID-19 pandemic, many people had to deal with yet another factor impacting skin health: the effects of prolonged use of face masks. Even though face masks might help skin stay younger by protecting the lower part of the face from UV radiation, overall it was found that the prolonged use of face masks contributes to acne[8] due to the repeated mechanical friction and irritation.[9]

In addition to the impact of certain environmental factors, skin aging may be accelerated by psychological stress and physical exhaustion resulting from lack of sleep.[10] Stress creates persistent muscle tension and can lead to chronic inflammation, which damages the skin's structure and creates wrinkles. Lack of sleep interferes with the skin's regeneration, and chronic sleeplessness increases the damage.

Smoking, excessive alcohol consumption, poor nutrition, and certain other lifestyle factors have also been shown to accelerate skin aging.[11] Women's skin is generally thinner and more vulnerable than men's skin, and it is therefore more sensitive to harmful environmental factors. After the age of fifty, women in or approaching menopause start

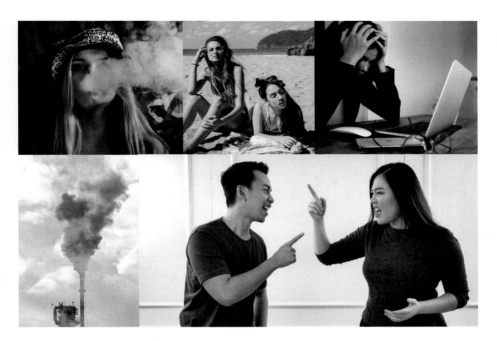

Figure I.2. Some detrimental factors that cause premature aging of the skin include: UV radiation, environmental toxins, stress, lack of sleep, poor nutrition, smoking, excessive alcohol consumption, negative emotions, and lack of exercise.

experiencing a decline in female sex hormones, which leads to decreased production of structural proteins in the skin and therefore more rapid aging of the skin compared to men. And as the load of environmental toxins we're exposed to on a daily basis seems to increase every year, it becomes more and more challenging to keep one's skin beautiful and vital, especially as women advance in age.

In the United States, the cosmetics industry is mostly self-regulated, while the pharmacology industry is regulated extensively and heavily. For a product to be considered a cosmetic (and therefore less regulated) and not a pharmacological product, it has to fit the following definition as established by the U.S. Food and Drug Administration: "The Federal Food, Drug & Cosmetic Act (FD&C Act) defines cosmetics as 'articles intended to be rubbed, poured, sprinkled, or sprayed on, introduced into, or otherwise applied to the human body for cleansing, beautifying, promoting attractiveness, or altering the appearance.'" And this is how U.S. law defines a pharmaceutical drug: "The FD&C Act defines drugs as 'articles intended for use in the diagnosis, cure, mitigation, treatment, or prevention of disease and articles (other than food) intended to affect the structure or any function of the body of man or other animals.'" Over-the-counter drugs are drugs that can be purchased without a doctor's prescription.

By these definitions, cosmetic products can cleanse, beautify, promote attractiveness, or alter one's appearance; however, they cannot repair, rejuvenate, prevent aging, and do most of the things people are buying them for. In other countries the regulations may be different; however in any country there are protective laws in place that are aimed at making cosmetic products safer while limiting what they can actually do to improve the skin.

If cosmetic products are not drugs and cannot, according to the legal definition established by the FDA, repair, rejuvenate, and regenerate skin, what *can* they do? Here is where we enter the gray area of "cosmeceutical" skin products, referring to the curious blend of the words *cosmetic* and *pharmaceutical*. Even though legally there is no such category as cosmeceuticals, many cosmetic companies take risks and include in their formulations biologically active compounds that can theoretically influence the biological processes in the skin. However, because by law cosmetic products are allowed only superficial, temporary, "cosmetic" effects, there is no way to verify whether the highly acclaimed "biologically active" ingredients in such formulations actually do what they are supposed to do. Many cosmetic companies use vague language to communicate to their customers many wonderful and desirable benefits of the supposedly biologically active ingredients in their products; however anyone attempting to figure out how much of a highly acclaimed herbal extract, peptide, mineral, or vitamin the product actually contains would not be able to do so, as this is closely guarded proprietary information.

The ideal skin-care product would help the skin look younger, protect it from damage, and make it appear more radiant and beautiful.

However, even the most advanced and expensive cosmetic product can only reach the very topmost layer of the skin. Because of the premium placed on beauty and youth, cosmetic skin-care is a multibillion-dollar industry, one that pours astronomical sums into advertising while sending women on a wild goose chase as they keep trying to find that special, revolutionary, advanced skin-care product that promises to erase wrinkles and turn back the clock. A glamorous young model, illuminated by carefully positioned lighting and featuring professionally applied makeup, looks out at us from the covers of women's magazines and internet pages, suggesting that anyone who buys the newest, most advanced, "scientifically proven and dermatologically tested" cosmetic product can achieve the same beautiful skin.

While so many of us chase the impossible dream of having eternally youthful, wrinkle-free skin, we may fail to realize that our skin is a living, breathing organ that possesses its own magic of healing, renewal, and rejuvenation. No skin-care product can ever replace our natural biological systems, which are best designed to do this job. Yes, it is

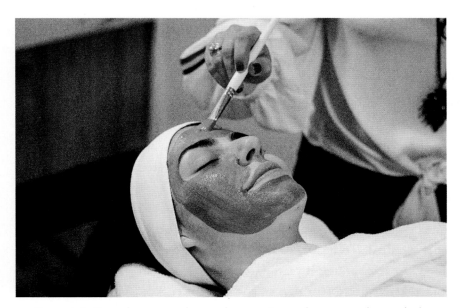

Figure I.3. Even the most advanced cosmetic product can only reach the topmost layer of the skin.

possible at any age to have beautiful, healthy, radiant, luminous skin. It is possible to have skin that perfectly expresses our inner beauty and radiance. To achieve this we must consider the internal needs of the skin, and not only its external, superficial qualities.

In the past, a good doctor could make an accurate diagnosis of a patient's health just by looking at their skin. A web of red, inflamed blood vessels on the skin's surface; a yellowish, bluish, or greenish tint; a pale complexion; bags under one's eyes; various spots and rashes—all these symptoms can be used to diagnose conditions of the internal organs. This is possible because the health and balance of every organ immediately affects the health and appearance of the skin. The skin is the body's largest organ; it covers the entire body and is exposed to the outside environment. It protects all the organs and defines a person's internal environment. This large and important organ has to be maintained, fed, oxygenated, hydrated, protected, repaired, and balanced. This is a big job, one that involves every organ and system in the body. The skin needs oxygen from the lungs, nutrients from the digestive system, protection by the immune system, and receives signals from the nervous and endocrine systems.

Many people understand the need to have balanced nutrition and the importance of detoxifying and exercising, along with practicing a quality skin-care routine. Yet nowadays there are so many diets, exercise programs, and nutritional supplements to support one's quest for health and youthful vigor that it's easy to become overwhelmed. Countless books promising rejuvenation and revitalization are out there, and often they offer conflicting advice. People try one system after another, only to end up feeling confused and unsatisfied. What is needed is a simple, logical, science-based, time-tested system that simultaneously improves one's emotional, physical, and spiritual well-being while restoring radiance, vitality, and beauty to the skin.

Over five thousand years ago in China, ancient Taoist masters who had a keen interest in nature and the inner workings of the human mind and body developed a philosophy that has been called the "original science." Taoism is not a religion. It is a spiritual discipline that anyone can practice. Through experimentation, observation, and diligent meditative practice, early Taoists were able to develop a surprisingly effective and powerful system of personal energy cultivation through the practice of Chi Kung, which allows a person to replenish their vital organs—including the skin—by focusing and directing the life force into them. For thousands of years, Taoist practices were kept secret and never taught to foreigners. Even when Eastern teachers started traveling to the West to teach Tai Chi, Kung Fu, and Chi Kung, most of them would only teach the external movements, without revealing the movements of the mind and the secrets of energy mastery.

The Universal Healing Tao system is designed to work with your body's own self-regulating and healing mechanisms. Without the knowledge of modern biochemistry, ancient Taoist masters developed practices of energy cultivation for health, vitality, and vibrancy, and these practices are increasingly being acknowledged by modern science. Today Taoist practices have helped hundreds of thousands of people heal from emotional and physical ailments, increase their vitality and sexual power, achieve more balance in life, boost their immune system, and strengthen their body and spirit. Medical research confirms the benefits of Chi Kung (also rendered *Qigong*) in the treatment of depression, arthritis, Parkinson's disease, and Type 2 diabetes, as well as in the rehabilitation of stroke and cancer patients.[12] A 2019 meta-analysis published in the *American Journal of Chinese Medicine* concluded that Chi Kung, when practiced at least three times a week, favorably influences physical ability, balance, and overall functioning in elderly adults.[13]

The main reason the Universal Healing Tao system developed by Master Chia is very effective at achieving more beautiful and radiant skin is because these practices work with the body's own self-regulating and healing mechanisms to address issues of renewal, detox, improved circulation and breathing, reduce stress and muscle tension, and restore the body to its optimal state. And this is exactly what is missing in the current skin-care industry. Many other types of practices make the mistake of focusing either solely on the physical body or disregarding the body entirely and focusing only on spiritual growth. Some extreme spiritual practices go as far as to advocate "mortifying" the flesh, i.e., beating the body into submission through pain, starvation, and hard work. The Tao teaches us to love our body and take good care of it, while cultivating energy and developing one's spiritual essence to achieve a state of happiness, pleasure, and delight.

For this book we selected energy practices that are generally considered safe. However, we advise you to carefully monitor your responses and take it easy. There should be no pain, dizziness, or any other unpleasant sensations. If you feel you need more guidance or would like to go deeper, we recommend finding a qualified Universal Healing Tao instructor to guide you through the practices.*

The authors of this book selected Taoist practices specifically tailored to enhance the skin's health and beauty. By putting the concepts and especially the exercises presented in this book into one's regular practice, you will gain a more radiant and uplifted appearance, a greater sense of personal confidence and beauty, a healthier and more youthful complexion, visible reduction of wrinkles, and an overall more attractive and luminous quality to your skin.

Thousands of years ago ancient Taoists discovered that our internal organs as well as the skin renew and rejuvenate from within. They developed powerful practices for balancing and awakening the body's innate wisdom and healing powers. Today, thanks to the discoveries of modern science, we know that the skin indeed has more potential for regeneration and renewal than was previously believed. Moreover, many signs of aging that in the past were attributed to the passage of time are now known to be signs of damage inflicted by external and internal factors. For example, it is now known that stress and negative emotions affect the skin even more than environmental toxins and UV radiation.[14]

Today, powerful technologies for balancing and renewal developed by Taoist masters over many centuries are receiving increasing recog-

---

*If you need help finding an instructor, please go to universaltaoinstructors.com.

nition from scientists and beauty experts. This means that we can tap into this ancient wisdom, now supported by today's scientific knowledge, to achieve a more radiant and healthy skin, a greater sense of self-confidence, and lasting beauty. These qualities can be cultivated and enhanced even at a very advanced age, such that women and men of any age can create more radiant beauty and healthier and younger-looking skin. The practices presented in this book will help you get better results than what is available from beauty products and procedures. True radiance comes from vitality, and vitality comes from the life force, or *chi*. By replenishing, balancing, and directing their chi, those who seek beauty and rejuvenation can recharge, replenish, and reclaim their beauty and confidence.

The great advantage of the Taoist approach to beautiful skin is that it does not require expensive products, procedures, and surgeries. It is the ultimate DIY (do-it-yourself) approach to beauty and rejuvenation; it can be practiced anywhere, at any time, by anyone who is willing to commit to doing the practices on a regular basis.

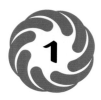

Beauty Is More than Skin-Deep

There is a Fountain of Youth: it is your mind, your talents, the creativity you bring to your life and the lives of the people you love. When you learn to tap this source, you will truly have defeated age.

SOPHIA LOREN

Every living organism on this planet, from a tiny insect to a majestic whale, has physical boundaries from the rest of the world around it. To be alive means to have a body that receives energy and resources from the outside environment while maintaining one's own sovereignty. This means that every living organism in the course of its evolution had to create some kind of a border that would allow for an energy exchange and interaction with its environment, yet would prevent the environment from invading the body. In all animals, including humans, this boundary is the skin. The skin divides the watery, warm, vulnerable inner environment of the body from the airy, dry, ever-changing, sometimes dangerous outer environment. Like the way a medieval castle had to have strong walls to protect its residents from hostile invaders, human skin needs to be strong and healthy to keep every organ safe and comfortable.

THE SKIN, A HOLISTIC VIEW

Skin is one of the most complex organs, and it deserves care and protection because of its essential role in a person's overall well-being. Culturally, the skin plays another role, which is also complex and not completely understood: it attracts people's attention and triggers powerful emotions. For women, especially, having smooth, radiant, blemish-free, slightly blushing skin is highly desirable and considered beautiful, whereas skin that is uneven, wrinkled, grayish, sagging, lifeless, inflamed, or blemished is not. This causes a lot of distress and unhappiness, even though eventually every person who lives a long time develops wrinkles and other signs of aging. Today, there is an increased number of people who respond to the societal pressure by refusing to conceal signs of aging.

Ironically, the attitude of being focused exclusively on one's external beauty is usually a major obstacle to maintaining the health and beauty of the skin. The Taoist approach to cultivating beautiful skin is holistic: it recognizes the skin's connection to all the major organs and every physiological process in the body, as well as the human mind, soul, and spirit. This is the only approach that restores the skin's health and beauty, and it all comes down to a relatively simple daily practice that does not require expensive creams and plastic surgery.

SKIN BEAUTY IS AN INSIDE JOB

Babies and young children have beautiful, smooth, plump, radiant skin. Most people think that the only reason why baby skin is so beautiful is because it's young. What they don't take into account is that babies and small children, before any kind of social conditioning, also have the most vibrant and unbound minds, souls, and spirits. A baby is born with abundant life force and energy that flows like a river, without any restrictions. By the time that being reaches adolescence, her skin starts to develop individuality. Some people notice their skin becoming thicker and oilier, while others notice their skin becoming thinner and more sensitive. In time, the skin will usually start displaying various forms of internal imbalance and external defects as a result of living life on this planet. By the age of thirteen, some people may still have beautiful, smooth, flawless skin, while others may start struggling with enlarged pores, blemishes, and oily sheen. Some people have only a few acne spots, while others may suffer from inflamed lesions, clogged pores, large patches of red skin, and acne scarring. Even at a relatively young age, young people become aware of their skin's imperfections and start searching for ways to improve their looks. Yet many do not realize that the weight of other people's opinions as well as one's personal insecurities and poor eating habits, too much time spent sitting down instead of playing outdoors, and suppressing one's creativity are among the many factors that have a tremendous impact on the skin's quality.

With age, individual differences in skin quality begin to emerge. While some people receive many compliments for their beautiful skin, others come to the conclusion that they are unattractive due in large part to the condition of their skin. One person may pass through their teenage years and never have a blemish, while another may continue to struggle with acne breakouts well into their forties and even beyond. Those who have skin like rose petals and fine silk may keep getting compliments and feel confident in their attractive appearance, and those who have blemishes or scarring may feel a lack of self-confidence and use a lot of makeup to conceal their flaws. Those who believe they are unattractive may develop various insecurities that would lead them to suppress their creativity and sacrifice themselves for others' sake, acquiring a high level of stress and anxiety in the process. They may comfort themselves with sugary food, alcohol, and other unhealthy habits in an effort to assuage their feelings of unattractiveness. All these factors impact the skin's health and radiance.

After the age of fifty, many women witness their skin begin to wrinkle as a result of hormonal changes, and some experience this as early as age forty. And for men and women regardless of their gender identity who have been blessed with a long life, there will come a time when the skin starts visibly aging despite all efforts. For those who have based their identity and self-esteem on their beautiful skin, this loss may cause great suffering. Since the skin is so intricately linked to one's self-expression, emotions, and overall health, everything that affects the mind, body, soul, and spirit will affect the skin.

As a physical structure, the human body slowly accumulates wear and tear, and the skin, as an organ that gets exposed to the outer elements, will eventually show signs of damage and deterioration. At the same time, though, it must be remembered that the human body has the capacity to renew, regenerate, and rebuild damaged tissues, including the skin. Today, the multibillion cosmetics industry continuously searches for methods and technologies to renew, regenerate, and rebuild aging skin, or at least help conceal damage. The main limitation of all cosmetic approaches, however, lies in the word *cosmetic,* which means "superficial." There is no cosmetic product in the world that can truly renew and rejuvenate the skin, because true renewal and rejuvenation must begin inside the body and must also include the mind, soul, and spirit.

In the West, people are used to going to an external authority to solve all their problems. They go to a doctor if they are sick, hire a lawyer to get a legal advice, take their car to a repair shop when it breaks down, and buy a cosmetic product when they need to improve their skin. The multibillion-dollar advertising industry has shaped people's minds and trained them to look outside of themselves for any and all solutions. However, very often when the body has reached a point where it needs a lot of external help, it is actually beyond help. The same is true for the skin. When the skin reaches the point when it needs help from a plastic surgeon, it will take a lot of money and effort to make it look young and beautiful.

Yet science is finally starting to recognize that skin beauty, just like the body's health and vitality, is an inside job. The human body, from the moment of conception to the moment of death, is well-equipped to balance hormones, absorb nutrients, remove toxins, and repair damage. Every cell in the body contains knowledge and wisdom that allows us to heal and regenerate. Yet modern life has disconnected people from their body's innate healing wisdom, and this has led us to unhappiness, early aging, and illness. Taoist practices for skin renewal allow us to get back to our body's own innate wisdom to restore our skin's regenerative powers. When we put the physical body, the mind, and the life force (chi) together, we can align with this power and awaken our intrinsic healing capabilities.

THE FUNCTIONS OF THE SKIN

Most people buy cosmetic products expecting them to do what they promise. The problem is, they don't. Here are some claims frequently made in skin-care marketing:

- Repairs past damage
- Delivers high levels of hydration
- Dramatically reduces visible signs of aging
- Reduces the look of every key sign of aging
- Frees skin from visible accumulation of excessive damage
- Promises fresh, new radiance every morning
- Firms and brightens up tired, slack skin
- Plumps sagging skin for a more lifted, firm, sculpted look

To anyone familiar with skin biology and functions, it is obvious that repairing past damage, delivering high levels of hydration, reducing the look of every key sign of aging, freeing the skin from the accumulation of excessive damage, firming, brightening, and so on requires much more than merely the application of creams and serums on the skin's surface layer. This is because the skin is a complex organ comprising different tissues. It is the body's largest organ, intimately connected to all the other organs and systems. Yet the skin-care industry, with its many promises, continues to entice people to buy their products because the skin is one of the most important biological features in our interactions and communications with others. Smooth, radiant, blemish-free, healthy, youthful-looking skin is a highly desirable, sought-after, envy-worthy attribute, one that so many people value and admire.

Yet the skin is more than just a beautiful wrapping for the body. The skin has a variety of functions:

- **Shielding from invaders:** The skin is a mechanical barrier protecting the body from intruders such as viruses and bacteria.
- **Preservation of moisture:** Without the skin, the body would dry out very fast. The skin consists of layers of complex, water-holding structures that make sure both the skin itself and the body it covers have enough moisture.
- **Thermoregulation:** The skin insulates the body and helps it release excess heat. Because of the skin, people can maintain a constant body temperature, even when the outside temperature fluctuates.
- **Sensation:** The skin is what touches the world and other living beings. The skin is what is being touched by the world and other living beings. The skin is what experiences the warmth of the sun and the coolness of a breeze. It's what itches when a child puts on a woolen sweater gifted by Grandma. It's what crawls at the sight of an unpleasant person. It's what tingles with delight at a lover's touch.
- **Regulation of endocrines:** The skin produces vitamin D when it is exposed to sunlight, and it also produces a host of biologically active compounds, including sex hormones. The skin is also responsive to hormones. It feels stress and other emotions.
- **Detoxification:** The skin is the largest detox organ in human body. It releases CO_2 and metabolic toxins through its many pores and detoxifies toxins through its antioxidant system.
- **Respiration:** Skin can absorb oxygen from the air and release CO_2.
- **Display of social cues:** For human beings, our skin is an essential and inevitable component of our beauty. The skin is impossible to ignore. It helps people express and communicate emotions, and it often betrays people by revealing their feelings, such as blushing or getting pale, perspiring, or getting goosebumps.
- **Exchange of energy:** The skin is an organ through which our personal energy radiates out into the world. Electromagnetic

energy, which radiates from the heart, has to pass through the physical boundary that is the skin. Energy that flows from a person's palms and fingertips is shaped and altered by the unique swirls and grooves on the person's skin. The skin also receives and transmits energy into the body. By regulating its tension, the skin can let more energy through or limit the amount of energy that comes in and out.

SKIN RENEWAL, THE KEY TO LASTING BEAUTY

The skin can perform all its many diverse functions and stay beautiful and radiant because it continuously renews itself. The same process that heals scrapes and cuts on a child's knee and elbow without leaving any signs of past damage works in every person's skin every day, repairing, renewing, rejuvenating, and maintaining the skin's integrity and functionality. Without daily regeneration, human beings would have aged, tattered, worn-looking skin within weeks of their first contact with the outside environment. Young, healthy skin renews itself with vigor and high efficiency. As people age, however, skin renewal slows down. Skin renewal is the key to lasting and radiant beauty, and this is why so many scientific studies are dedicated to studying its mechanisms. To harness the magic of skin renewal is to harness the magic of rejuvenation.

At the heart of skin renewal are special cells called *stem cells,* the body's raw materials from which it can create new skin cells and which can transform into blood vessel cells, nerve cells, connective tissue cells, fat cells, brain cells, muscle cells, and so on. In the skin alone there are three main groups of stem cells: epidermal stem cells, located in the lower layer of the epidermis; hair follicle stem cells, located in the bulge region of hair follicles; and mesenchymal stem cells, located in subcutaneous fat. Because the skin is organized in various layers, with each layer having its own structure and renewal schedule, most people never notice the process of skin renewal that occurs continu-

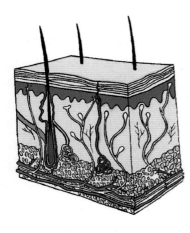

epidermis

dermis

subcutaneous fat

Figure 1.1.
The skin consists of
three layers as seen in
this cross section.

ously because the skin can repair itself without anyone noticing. The only time we become aware of skin regeneration is when our skin is wounded, burned, or injured in some way that disrupts its integrity. Depending on the size and depth of an injury, the skin can heal completely and without any residual damage, or it can develop scars, redness, ulcers, and other complications. Many cosmetic procedures, such as chemical peels, microneedling, lasers, and dermabrasion, work by either triggering inflammation or by applying controlled damage to trigger a robust regeneration response. Unfortunately, such procedures may result in skin damage and accelerated aging.[1]

The skin consists of three layers, all of which are renewable: the epidermis, the dermis, and a layer of subcutaneous fat.

The Epidermis

The most active and vigorously renewed layer of the skin is the epidermis, the outermost layer, which is itself further divided into distinct layers. When all layers of the epidermis are renewed properly and without delay, the skin looks smooth, radiant, and beautiful. The epidermis is only 0.04–1.5 millimeters thick. Its bottommost layer, located on the border with the dermis, contains small, round, slowly dividing stem cells that sit on a special structure called the *basal membrane.* This is a foundational structure that provides a stable surface for the epidermal stem cells. The epidermal stem cells remain small, round, and uniform as long as they are attached to the basal membrane. Once a new skin cell leaves the safety of its birthplace it cannot stop its journey; it will grow, mature, and move up to the surface. While an epidermal skin cell moves up to the outermost surface of the skin, it becomes bigger and starts accumulating a protein called *keratin.* Eventually all of the cell's interior is replaced by keratin, and the cell flattens. By the time these skin cells reach the surface layer, called the *stratum corneum,* they are no longer alive.

The entire surface of the skin is covered with layers of these dead cells that no longer look like cells. They are thin, flat, translucent, cornified cells (corneocytes, or keratinous scales). Each scale is 20–40 microns wide and 0.5 of a micron thick. In healthy skin, all keratinous scales are glued together by lipids and form a kind of flexible armor. When this upper layer is healthy and smooth and well-hydrated, the skin looks radiant, smooth, and youthful. For the stratum corneum, the skin's surface, to be so smooth, healthy, and well-hydrated, the whole epidermis has to renew regularly. A young epidermis renews itself in just two to three weeks,[2] which is why babies and children easily heal from wounds and other skin injuries and do not need moisturizers or antiwrinkle creams.

Skin renewal slows down with age, and after age forty it can take four to six or more weeks to renew the entire epidermis. At this point the skin surface is starting to lose its smoothness and luster. This is when moisturizing creams that fill the upper layers of the skin with water and add liveliness and radiance can be useful. Since pollution and other damaging factors alter the protein structure inside the scales that form the outermost layer of the skin, environmental conditions can make the skin look dull and cloudy, which in turn creates a more aged and tired expression. This is why creams for daytime use containing UV filters and antioxidants can be so useful in slowing down the signs of skin aging. When the skin is well-moisturized, it becomes better at reflecting and transmitting light. It is also better at transmitting electromagnetic energy (this actually can be measured). When the skin is dry, its keratinous scales shrink and become rough and uneven. As a result, the skin loses its radiance. And when the skin does not glow, every blemish, every wrinkle, and every imperfection becomes more visible.

Even though cosmetic products can greatly help to brighten, uplift, and enliven the skin, they create only a temporary improvement, for true replenishment and rejuvenation has to start much deeper. Taoist energy-moving meditations found in various Chi Kung practices address the key issue of fading beauty due to slower skin renewal. By working on all the organs and tissues, including the skin, these practices help tap into the skin's own renewal potential and so can reverse many of the effects of ongoing skin damage and aging.

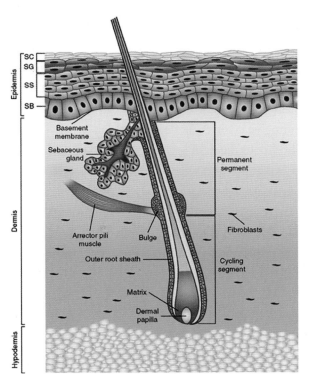

Figure 1.2. Location of stem cells in the skin.
Creative commons illustration as seen in D. J. Wong and H. Y. Chang, "Skin Tissue Engineering," (March 31, 2009), StemBook, ed. The Stem Cell Research Community, doi/10.3824/stembook.1.44.1

The Dermis

The epidermis is supported by the much thicker dermis. While the epidermis is comprised of layers of cells, the dermis has much fewer cells. Unlike the epidermis, the dermis has nerves and blood vessels. This layer resembles a mattress; it has "springs" made from resilient proteins (collagen and elastin) and it has the "stuffing" of gel-like matter composed of large molecules of glycosaminoglycan. Collagen and elastin form the supporting structure, which in young people keeps the skin supple, smooth, and resilient. With age, the protein structures become weaker and worn-out, so the skin starts sagging and develops wrinkles.

Fortunately the dermis has its own master builders, called *fibroblasts.* These cells continuously renew and repair worn-out skin structures and break down old collagen and elastin, replacing them with brand-new collagen and elastin. Fibroblasts also renew and replenish a special gel made from glycosaminoglycan that consists of large polymer molecules that fill the space between the collagen and the elastin "springs," creating skin firmness and the soft, sumptuous appearance of youthful skin. Children have plenty of glycosaminoglycan in their dermis, which is why their cheeks are so plump and fresh-looking. Collagen, elastin, and fibroblasts are all immersed in this water-holding gel, so when glycosaminoglycan starts breaking down and diminishes with age, the dermis starts losing its supportive qualities.

Unless the dermis is renewed and regenerated it is impossible to achieve beautiful skin. The dermis gives skin its resilience, elasticity, suppleness, radiance, and glow. Unfortunately, most cosmetic products never reach the dermis. To some extent the volume of the dermis can be restored by injecting special skin-plumping polymers such as hyaluronic acid, collagen, and artificial gels; however, they only restore the volume but not the glow and freshness of young skin. To replenish the dermis, the skin has to break down its old collagen and elastin and manufacture new collagen and elastin, repair and regenerate blood vessels and nerves, and replace the water-holding gel regularly. Taoist Chi Kung practices work with the skin's blood vessels, nerves, lymph, and water balance, while stimulating stem cells for a younger regenerated state.

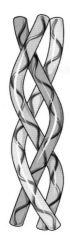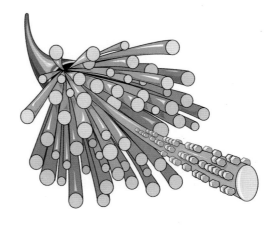

Figure 1.3. LEFT: Collagen, with its triple helix, and elastin make the dermis firm, smooth, and resilient. RIGHT: A microscopic cross-section of a piece of the helix is shown.

The Subcutaneous Fat Layer

The bottommost layer of subcutaneous fat has the slowest renewal rate. This layer is important because it shapes the face and body, provides insulation, and cushions against mechanical insults, protecting internal organs and skin. The fatty layer also contains blood vessels and is closely connected to underlying skin muscles. When the cheeks and under-eye areas start losing their fatty layer, the result is a characteristic hollow look, which creates a tired and aged appearance. The subcutaneous fat layer has its own stem cells, and so it too can be renewed. The renewal rate depends on many factors, including the state of the blood vessels and the level of toxins in the skin. One thing is for sure: there is very little that cosmetic products can do to restore the layer of subcutaneous fat. One approach has been to inject a person's own fat cells into facial skin to replace lost volume. Another is to seed the subcutaneous fat with fresh stem cells and hope they will stimulate renewal. There are also various types of deep tissue massage, vibratory massagers for the face, and the injection of biologically active compounds into the skin, called *mesotherapy.* All these procedures are costly, often invasive, and have limited success. They also have to be repeated because the skin continues to age. Fortunately fatty tissue has its own powerful renewal resource, the mesenchymal stem cells. These cells possess an amazing restorative potential and are now being actively studied by medical researchers as a potential treatment for many types of ailments.

Chi Kung practices are perfectly suited for activating stem cells in the fatty tissues. Chi Kung masters apply the vibrational force of bamboo hitters and other tactics to loosen up the fat and encourage better blood flow, better lymph drainage, and better regeneration.

COSMETIC ILLUSIONS VERSUS TRUE RENEWAL

Young skin looks so warm and alive. Yet even in young skin there are structures that technically are not alive. These structures become a common target for cosmetic products and procedures as we mature because they are so easy to alter. It takes weeks to renew, rebuild, and rejuvenate the skin naturally, while it takes only seconds to alter it mechanically by changing the level of hydration in its "dead" structures. As described above, the very upper layer of the skin, its stratum corneum, or horny layer, is composed entirely of dead cells that are thin, flat, hard, translucent scales filled with the protein keratin. Keratin is the same protein from which fingernails, hair, hooves, and horns are made—which is why the upper layer of the skin is called "the horny layer."

Keratinous scales on the skin's surface have no nucleus and no cell membranes; they do not feed or grow, and after they are worn out they shed and become dust. This is why the upper layer of the skin can be safely saturated with water, which causes the stratum corneum to swell, creating a quite believable illusion of rejuvenation. To create such an illusion, cosmetic products may contain detergents that temporarily make the stratum corneum more permeable. If it's done briefly and delicately, this is not a problem. However, such methods too often can eventually make the skin more vulnerable to irritants and other potentially toxic substances. After all, the stratum corneum is designed to prevent water from getting in or out of the skin.

Most cosmetic creams contain emollients, oily substances that temporarily make the stratum corneum softer and smoother. Many modern emollients are chemically altered oils that are quite foreign to the skin. Another way to make the skin appear younger is by creating a polymer film on it, which tightens and uplifts the skin. Ingredients such as acrylate copolymers serve this purpose. Needless to say, they provide a quick fix to assuage one's vanity, but do little to help the skin renew itself.

Another desirable target for cosmetic products is the dermis. Even though cosmetic ingredients cannot reach it, there are still ways to affect the conditions of the soft glycosaminoglycan gel in the dermis. The dermal matrix holds a space for the skin's structural proteins such as collagen and elastin, which support the skin and make it plump and resilient. The dermal matrix receives hydration from its blood vessels; however the epidermis does not have its own blood vessels and depends on the water that migrates from the dermis. In healthy skin there is a balance between the water that evaporates from the skin's surface and the water that comes from the dermis. Anything that creates an effect of occlusion and reduces the amount of water loss from the surface will increase

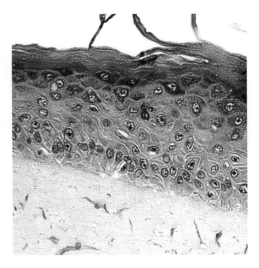

Figure 1.4. The swelling of the stratum corneum (seen nearest the top of the image) creates an immediate effect of rejuvenation.

hydration of the dermis. Therefore, cosmetic products and procedures that temporarily block water loss from the surface would tend to create plumper, more youthful-looking skin.

Every cosmetic product is designed with the goal of making the skin look younger, softer, smoother, more luminous, and, of course, more beautiful. This is why cosmetic chemists focus first and foremost on creating an effect that the buyer will notice immediately. This is how cosmetic products are marketed. A potential buyer is offered a cream or serum to try on their skin. The product has a nice smell (which means it contain fragrances, often artificial); can sit on a cosmetic counter in an open tester without going bad (which means it contains preservatives); and feels soft and nice (which means it contains emollients). When applied, it immediately transforms the skin, creating a plumper, tighter, more lifted, and much smoother complexion. There are also cosmetic products that contain biologically active ingredients and actually help the skin stay healthier and more radiant. A typical modern cosmetic product is a marvel of chemistry. Its list of ingredients may contain emollients, petroleum jelly, silicones, texture adjusters, emulsifiers, film-forming polymers, preservatives, fragrance, chemical dyes, and just a wee bit of biologically active substances.

However it is important to understand that for the cosmetics industry the inclusion of biologically active ingredients is not a high priority, because the skin is a living tissue, and real rejuvenating effects from quality skin-care may take up to two to six weeks to appear. Unfortunately in many cases the need to create a product that has a long shelf-life, a pleasant smell, spreads easily, and absorbs in seconds to make the skin immediately smoother and softer usually means a chemical nightmare for the skin, since it has to deal with dozens of chemical substances that can irritate it, disturb its integrity, cause allergic reactions, or alter its own chemistry. Most cosmetic products nowadays are much safer than they used to be due to rigorous testing and higher standards for safety; however, there are more subtle influences that may not necessarily cause immediate harm but may weaken the skin's ability to renew itself.

SKIN RENEWAL NEEDS ENERGY

Unlike other organs such as the liver or the brain, the skin is not easy to weigh; nevertheless its weight has been calculated. Presently the estimated weight of the skin for an average adult is between nine and twenty pounds, and the total skin surface is about twenty to twenty-two square feet.[3] In healthy young skin, the epidermis completely renews itself every two weeks. This means that with a two-week renewal rate, the body has to have enough energy to renew twenty to twenty-two square feet of skin every two weeks! No wonder renewal takes longer and longer as people age and as energy becomes depleted. By the age of forty, skin renewal takes four to six weeks, while at the age of seventy it can slow down to eight to ten weeks.[4]

One of the reasons why skin regeneration slows down when we age is because many stem cells have become dormant—they stop listening to signals from other cells and remain inactive instead of repairing the skin. To awaken the skin's regenerative ability, its "sleeping beauty" has to be awakened. One way to do this is by using peeling agents such as alpha-hydroxy acids, which inflict mild damage on the skin's surface, forcing stem cells to wake up and repair the skin. However if there is not enough energy to support regeneration, not enough blood flow to deliver oxygen and nutrients, and more toxins than the skin can safely tolerate, such mild damage will not produce the desired result and may even cause further irritation, excessive pigmentation, and scarring.

BEYOND SKIN ANATOMY AND SKIN AS A WHOLE

Western anatomy is valuable because it allows us to understand how various methods of skin rejuvenation work. Yet it is also a hindrance because it breaks what is essentially a unified whole down into discreet parts, and separate parts do not exist in nature. Skin, with its layers of epidermis, dermis, and subcutaneous fat, works as one holistic system that interacts with all the other organs of the body. The subcutaneous fat layer provides a soft and firm pillow and shapes the body so the dermis layer has some support. Without the underlying cushioning of fat, the dermis would not be able to function. The dermis supplies moisture, nutrients, and structural support to a much thinner epidermis. The epidermis protects all layers with its renewable stratum corneum made of cells that are no longer alive and can therefore withstand harsh conditions. And yet even this more integrated view must also include the entire body, as the skin rests on a layer of muscle and fascia, which in turn is connected to the bone structure. Blood is pumped by the heart and has to flow through the lungs to receive oxygen and pass through the intestines to get nutrients, and through the liver and kidneys to detox. Every tissue in the body is regulated by the nervous and endocrine systems and protected by the immune system.

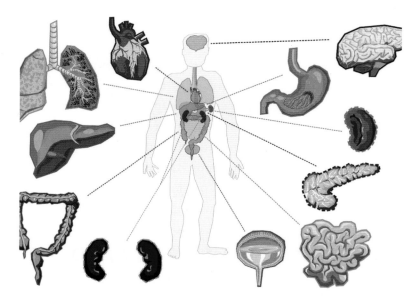

Figure 1.5. The skin's beauty and vitality depend on every organ in the body. The lungs supply oxygen and remove CO_2; the heart pumps blood to bring oxygen and nutrients to skin cells and remove CO_2 and toxic waste; the liver and kidneys detox blood; the nervous and endocrine systems regulate the skin's metabolism and renewal; the immune system protects the skin from viruses, bacteria, and foreign matter; and the musculoskeletal system supports and moves the skin.

There is also a strong emotional component to the skin. For example, people who are depressed and dispirited look very different from those who are inspired and enlightened. There is a wealth of sensations that come from the skin and to the skin. The feeling of warm raindrops on the skin will trigger a different chemical reaction within the skin neurology than the feeling of a blustery wind. Rays of warm sunshine may be dangerous because of the UV radiation they emit, yet they also can be healing because of the sense of comfort they create. The truth is that it's quite impossible to understand the skin from a strictly anatomical, physiological, or chemical perspective. Even the effects of cosmetic products and procedures can be different depending on a person's energy level, mood, personal circumstances, and beliefs. One person can walk into a cosmetic salon and walk out after receiving a treatment with glowing, radiant skin, while another person getting the same treatment, administered by the same person, may be covered in red blotches and develop other complications.

So since the skin is much more than the sum of its cells or anatomical parts, in reality we can say that beauty is more than skin-deep.

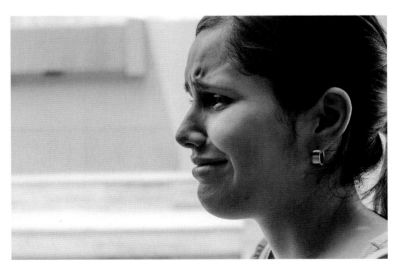

Figure 1.6. The skin is responsive to emotional and physical states of being. Worry and stress create wrinkles and diminish the skin's radiance.

Just as a person cannot achieve radiant health only as a result of taking pharmaceutical drugs and getting surgery, the skin requires a whole mind/body/soul/spirit approach to be beautiful. Taoism goes back thousands of years and was developed with the understanding that the human being is an integrated, holistic system. Chi Kung involves training the entire organism to consciously direct one's chi, or life-force energy, and its practices are aimed at returning the whole body to balance and harmony. As an integral part of the body, the skin greatly benefits from these practices, which will in turn reward the practitioner with beauty, radiance, and deep comfort.

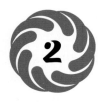

Taoist Secrets of Vitality and Vibrancy

One of the most noticeable qualities of young, healthy skin is its feeling of aliveness. This is the result of an abundant, free-flowing life force. No matter how carefully the skin is painted with cosmetics and no matter how smooth and tight it is, without that sense of energetic aliveness there is no beauty.

Every cell in the body needs energy. Every muscle. Every chemical reaction. The human body can only function optimally if it has sufficient energy in the form of electricity flowing through it. There is often a dramatic scene in movies that is set in a hospital room, where a heart monitor shows the peaks and valleys of a patient's heartbeat on a screen. When it flatlines, nurses and doctors run into the room and try to jumpstart the heart with powerful electrical shocks from a defibrillator. What shows on the heart monitor are electrical currents generated by cells in the heart. Every living cell produces such electricity and runs on electricity. Like the heart, without a supply of electromagnetic energy the skin cannot function, and it certainly cannot renew and regenerate.

RENEWING THE SKIN WITH ENERGY

Long before the advent of the scientific method, Taoists concluded that all living organisms have an innate ability to heal and balance themselves. There is no need to go to school to learn how to breathe, because the body knows how to breathe and deliver oxygen to every cell. Similarly, there is no need to go to medical school to learn how to use your heart, because the heart knows how to pump blood throughout the body. The body also knows how to balance chemicals and how to make the chemical compounds that are needed to renew its tissues. Because the skin, like the rest of the body, has the capacity to self-regulate and heal, it is important to know how to help this complex system function optimally and how to avoid disrupting its balance.

Ancient Taoist masters were the original scientists. Unlike modern scientists who believe they have to take things apart and break them down into discreet parts in order to study them, Taoists studied things as they are in life—as an interconnected whole. They observed a flowing river and noticed that its water had an abundant and strong flow and tasted sweet and fresh. They studied a stagnant pond and observed that its water tasted foul and unpleasant, and that it lacked the freshness and vibrancy of the river. In the same way, it seemed to them that young, healthy people were more like a flowing river, while sick, old ones resembled a stagnant pond. Taoists concluded that there must be something flowing through the body to animate and enliven it. This force cannot be seen, yet it is just as real in its manifestations as the wind that creates the movement of trees and grasses or the rippling of water on a pond.

Taoist masters of old developed a mind-body healing technology based on their observations and inner sensing; it allowed them to observe and study the effects of this vital force, called *chi,* in the body. Today modern science knows chi to be electromagnetic energy, the force that animates all living things and creates movement and flow in nature. A human body generates and uses bioelectricity, which obeys the same laws of nature as other forms of electromagnetic energy. Taoist masters deduced that just like wood can be burned to create fire, which in turn radiates light and heat, a human body must have some mechanism by which it burns biological matter to create the living fire that is chi, which warms the body and illuminates it from the inside. This is very much like burning wood, but in this case this process occurs in a more peaceful and controlled manner, through a series of chemical reactions.

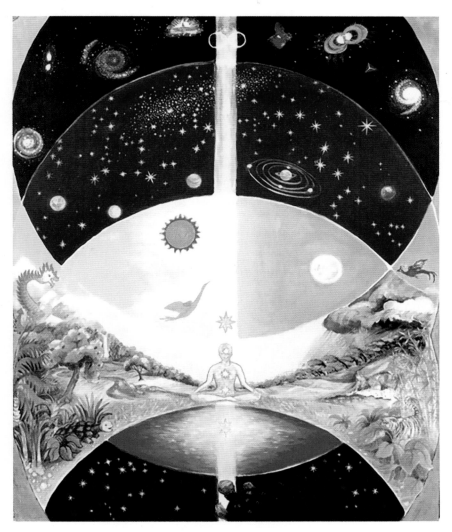

Figure 2.1. Ancient Taoists discovered the movements of chi in nature by observing flowing water, the wind, fire, sun and the planets, as well as plants and animals.

Taoist sages placed a premium on maintaining and protecting their chi. In young people, chi is bright and strong, shining through their eyes, illuminating their skin, and giving power to their thoughts and emotions. In older people it has clearly diminished, causing lifelessness, sluggishness, coldness of the body, and coldness of the emotions. So mastering the flow of chi means mastering the secrets of vitality and vibrancy. Over thousands of years of observation, practice, and experimentation, Taoist masters developed a powerful system of internal energy cultivation called *Chi Kung.**

Beauty Chi Kung is specifically focused on supporting and maintaining the vibrant flow of chi through the skin. When the flow of chi is restored, the skin will return to balance through its self-regulatory and self-balancing mechanisms. In some cases the skin may need additional help. However, no matter what pharmacological or cosmetic remedies are used and what surgical or technological procedures are performed, the skin can only renew and restore itself to its full vitality when it has enough chi.

CULTIVATING CHI

If you want to improve the flow of chi through your skin you have to realize that the skin's energy flow is not separate from the entire body's energy flow. In a human body, living cells receive most of their energy through a process called *oxidative phosphorylation*. This occurs in the cellular power stations, the mitochondria, which require oxygen to produce energy. With age, mitochondrial function starts declining, and this leads to increased formation of damaging free radicals, which are reactive atoms produced by certain biological processes or introduced from an outside source such as tobacco smoke, toxins in food, or any number of environmental pollutants. Free radicals can damage cells, proteins, and DNA by altering their chemical structure. Some methods of restoring the skin's energy function involve the use of coenzyme Q10

---

*_Chi_ means "energy"; _kung_ means "work."

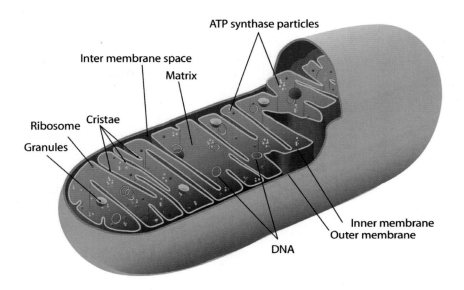

Figure 2.2. The mitochondria are the power stations inside cells.

(CoQ10) and creatinine, two nutrients that help the mitochondria generate energy in aging skin. Antioxidants such as ascorbic acid (vitamin C) have also been proven useful in preventing free-radical damage and delaying skin aging. The Taoist method involves restoring the energy flow to the skin through a whole-body, integrative approach.

In the Taoist tradition, the human body actually consists of three bodies: the physical body, the energy body, and the spiritual body (sometimes called the information body). As seen in figure 2.3 (p. 36), the Tao teaches that the physical, energetic, and spiritual bodies are not separate and exist in a continuous interplay with one another.

The Physical Body

The physical body is defined by its most exterior element, the skin. Everything that exists beyond the boundary that is the skin is not part of the physical body. For example, hair, even though it grows outside of the skin, is still considered part of the skin, whereas makeup and

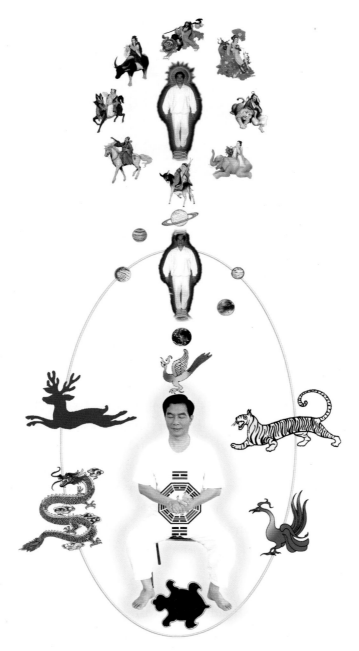

Figure 2.3. The three bodies of Taoism: the physical body (bottom), the energy body (middle), and the spiritual body (upper).

clothing obviously are not part of the skin and belong to the outside environment. The physical body is comprised of physical structures such as atoms, molecules, cells, tissues, and organs, which all obey the laws of nature. One such law is that of entropy, which states that all physical systems eventually lose energy and break down. All living organisms, including humans, have developed mechanisms to counteract entropy by repairing damaged structures and replenishing lost energy.

Theoretically, the human body could be immortal and remain eternally young if it had unlimited supplies of energy and an unlimited capacity to repair itself. Realistically, however, there are genetically determined limits on cellular renewal. This is known as the *Hayflick limit*. In 1961, American scientist Leonard Hayflick observed that cells in a culture can divide only forty to sixty times until they become senescent and start dying out. Since then, scientists have discovered that human cells can divide over a much longer period of time provided they have the right conditions. For example, human stem cells can be revived and rejuvenated even after they become senescent and stop dividing by supplying them with certain soluble growth factors derived from young tissue cells.[1]

In certain spiritual traditions the physical body is considered a burden, one that stifles the spirit and leads it into temptation. This is to not recognize the three bodies and their interdependence within the human organism. The ancient Taoist masters, with their scientific approach to life, discovered that the physical body can be viewed as a sophisticated device for transforming energy. It takes oxygen and nutrients from the outside environment and uses them to generate energy, which in turn can be used to replenish and regenerate the body's physical structures so that they can continue taking oxygen and nutrients in and thereby generate more energy. By paying close attention to how energy is generated and transformed, Taoists were able to develop surprisingly effective practices for restoring the body's vitality and therefore its beauty.

A Taoist practitioner learns to closely observe their own body to become familiar with the sensation of chi flowing through it and to cultivate what the body needs to keep it flowing. The skin needs oxygen and nutrients, hydration, and protection from harmful environmental influences, as well as the physical support provided by muscles and bones. It does not need the forty-some chemicals found in the average modern skin care product, which are used to make the product look, smell, and feel nice, and therefore easier to market. What the skin really needs is a clean and nourishing environment for the entire body to thrive so that the cells can function as they should.

The Energy Body

This is chi, the bioelectromagnetic energy generated by the cells in a physical organism that is needed in order to thrive and regenerate. The energy that moves through the body is expressed outwardly through the skin. When someone is in love or inspired, their skin shines; conversely, when someone is scared or depressed, their skin looks grayish and dull. The relationship between the physical body and the energy body can be understood through the metaphor of a lamp. Every lamp uses the same electromagnetic energy. And every lamp, depending on its structure, shines its light differently. The light can extend well beyond the boundaries of the lamp, but it still originates in the lamp, which is fed by a power source or a battery that delivers the electromagnetic energy to the lamp.

In the human body, electromagnetic energy has to be generated by physical structures that have channels or "wires" that allow the energy to flow and animate the body and the skin. These biological channels are known as the meridians in Traditional Chinese Medicine. In the Taoist tradition, now supported by quantum physics, the human energy body is connected to a much larger energy body, that of planet Earth, and to the even bigger energy body that is the entire universe. Since the same electromagnetic energy flows through everything in the universe and animates it, it can be taken into the body, processed, and then transformed into the body's own energy supply. The amount of energy the body can receive from breathing and eating food is limited, but the amount of energy the body can receive from other energy sources is potentially unlimited. In the past, there were no modern computers and internet, so the ancient masters had a hard time explaining the concept of interconnected energy. Today people are connecting to one another through Wi-Fi, so the idea of transmitting and receiving energy over any distance is no longer so foreign.

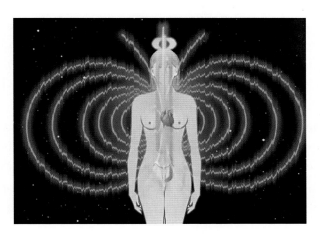

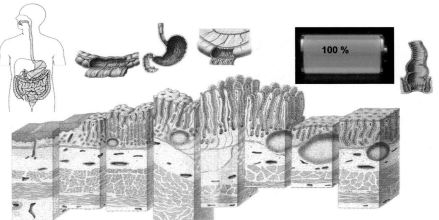

Figure 2.4. The physical body, which receives energy from oxygen, food, and the surrounding energy in the environment, serves as a kind of biobattery that generates electromagnetic energy. This energy radiates through the skin and connects to the energy of other living beings, nature, and the universe.

The Spiritual Body

The spiritual body includes human consciousness, which is also referred to as the mind, soul, and spirit. While the physical body is limited in what it can do and how much energy it can generate, the mind, soul, and spirit can reach the moon and the stars, travel into the past and into the future, and even reach into spiritual realms. The truth is, even the most prominent scientists cannot give a full explanation of what human consciousness is and where it comes from. It is confirmed, however, that the skin, with its many cells and nerves, responds to the movement of human consciousness. For example someone who is stuck in a soul-sucking job or whose spirit is crushed by devastating news or a painful breakup will often experience a loss of skin radiance, vitality, and beauty. No makeup or cosmetics can conceal the signs of despair, deep grief, or extreme exhaustion, and to be beautiful the skin requires a replenished physical body, a recharged and flowing bioelectromagnetic energy, and a vibrant spiritual body. The good news is that the energy practices of the Tao help restore energy flow on all these levels.

THE MIND-BODY CONNECTION

All organs, including the skin, work together because they are connected through our inner energetic "wiring" through which bioelectricity flows. In all organs and tissues, living cells generate electricity and magnetic fields. In animals, including humans, organs can communicate with high efficiency because they are all connected through specialized cells called *neurons*. Every neuron has a body and long tentacles called *axons* and *dendrites*. Axons and dendrites from individual neurons are bundled together in the cable-like structures that are the nerves. It is important to know that within every nerve, bundles of nerve fibers are wrapped in protective layers of connective tissue and fat. They also have fluid that's similar to spinal and cerebral fluid. This fluid has to move in order to keep the nerves supple and nourished.

Even though feelings and thoughts and other information transmitted through the nerves could be considered nonphysical, there are physical structures that support the flow of information. When neurons connect, they connect through a gap between their axons and dendrites, where they release neurochemicals. These neurochemicals affect more than the transmission of electrical impulse; they increase or decrease pain and inflammation and influence immune function and blood flow. Therefore any time nerve tissue is activated, chemical and physiological reactions are produced. Chi Kung practitioners learn to use these characteristics of the nervous system to increase vitality in the body by intentionally directing the flow of nerve impulses through the body. This is done by focusing and directing one's mind power.

Today, science has confirmed that focused attention allows people to direct the movement of electromagnetic energy through their

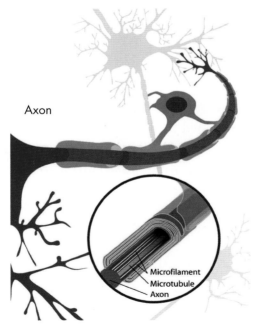

Figure 2.5. A nerve is like an electrical cable in which nerve fibers are bundled together and surrounded by protective layers of connective tissue and fat called *myelin*.

body—something that Taoist masters have been teaching for ages.[2] In other words, thoughts are not separate from the body and can be used to move electromagnetic energy to the tissues and organs.

The human brain has approximately 86 billion neurons. Out of this, 16 billion are in the newer and most human part of the brain, the neocortex; the rest comprise a much more ancient and primal structure. All neurons generate electromagnetic waves, which can be measured with an EEG machine. Modern science has discovered that in addition to the main brain located inside the skull there is another brain located in the abdominal area that has been called the "gut brain"; this is the enteric nervous system.[3] This abdominal brain is comprised of billions of neurons in the intestines that, like the main brain, can form memories and respond to various stimuli, including our thoughts. In fact, there is growing evidence that all the major organs, including the heart, harbor some kind of intelligence that can be developed and used to improve one's health and vitality.

Most modern people go to school so they can learn how to use their neocortex. Today it is very rare to meet someone who doesn't know how to speak, read, and write. However most people never really learn how to use their subcortical structures and the "body brains" located in the organs. This gap has been addressed in the ancient practices developed by Taoist masters, who dedicated thousands of years to studying the body's intelligence. The reason Taoist practices are so valuable for maintaining radiance, vitality, and beauty is because they work with energy and the intelligence found in all the major organs, including the skin.

TAOIST SECRETS OF ENERGY CULTIVATION

An esoteric principle says, "As above, so below." The same laws that govern the universe govern our body. Beauty and vibrancy of skin and body is created by the same mechanisms as what creates the beauty of blossoming flowers, flowing rivers, and lush, green forests. Like the way a stagnant river can be cleaned and restored to its natural flow, like the way depleted soil can be regenerated, or like the way fuel can be added to a campfire to create a brighter flame, it is possible to create more vibrancy and beauty for the skin and the rest of the body by replenishing and restoring its life force. But if we do nothing, our physical body will obey the law of entropy and keep on aging, deteriorating, and falling apart. Eventually, the river of life will dry out.

Taoist masters were very aware of the tendencies of entropy, and this is why they developed techniques for replenishing, recharging, restoring, and reactivating the flow of energy. For thousands of years they experimented, observed, and developed their practices. And they succeeded. Since earliest times Taoist masters have been legendary for their youthful appearance and their amazing agility and power, even at a very advanced age. Without knowing anything about bioelectricity and without having a modern knowledge of anatomy, physiology, and neuroscience, they found the recipe for the activation and restoration of the life force. Their practices include meditation and mindful movements for energy cultivation, which is the basis of the practice of Chi Kung, an ancient method that is way ahead of modern science.

Today we are witnessing an amazing merging of two worlds, the East and the West, since finally Western science has started to study and investigate the claims and practices of Chi Kung, giving fresh new support to this ancient knowledge. In order for the skin to regenerate and replenish itself, have a beautiful glow and a sumptuous, soft feel, it has to have enough energy. When energy is depleted, the skin suffers. Bioelectromagnetic energy is the golden river of chi that flows through all the cells, infusing them with radiance and vibrancy. This glow emanates from the skin, making it appear radiant and beautiful. For the electromagnetic energy from individual cells to merge into a unified flow of electricity throughout the entire body, there has to be a form of wiring through the body that traverses every tissue and every organ. In the human body this wiring is created by the nerves and the blood and lymphatic vessels, which, like the electrical wires and pipes in a modern building, carry oxygen, nutrients, and subtle information throughout the body.

THE SKIN'S NERVES AS CHANNELS FOR ENERGY

The skin has feelings. Hot and cold, pressure and stretching, gentle stroking, the touch of an annoyingly itchy sweater, splashes of water, the gentle breath of the wind, the warm rays of the sun, a silky garment, a lover's kiss; these are all detected and transmitted from the skin to the brain and to other organs through the many sensory nerves that traverse the dermis. The skin is innervated by cutaneous nerves that branch out from the spinal cord. Facial nerves also branch out from the trigeminal nerve from the brain stem. Each branch, which is called a *dermatome,* serves an area of the skin. To understand how complex skin innervation is, let's look at the different types of sensory units that provide such a richness of sensation:

Free nerve endings for C-fibers: These nerves, which lie very close to the surface of the skin, do not have myelin wrappings. They are extremely sensitive to chemical stimulation and to the slightest superficial touch. For example, they can detect an insect crawling over the skin or an irritating substance. If overstimulated, they release chemicals that cause inflammation and itching. Most cases of irritation from cosmetic products are caused by these nerves, which can also contribute to the inflammation associated with acne and make it worse. C-fibers become more sensitive if a person is stressed or emotionally upset. This accounts for the worsening of skin conditions during stress.

Merkel's disks: These are specialized receptors for touch and pressure. A lover's touch, massage, acupressure, or uncomfortable garments activate these nerves.

Miessneris corpuscles: These nerve endings are found in the hands and feet, and they respond to touch and pressure.

Mucocutaneous corpuscles: These are special receptors found only in mucous membranes such as inside the mouth or in the vagina.

Pacinian corpuscles: These are specialized receptors in the breasts and genitalia, as well as in deeper parts of the dermis of the palms and fingers and near the bones. They respond to pressure and vibration.

Pilo-Ruffini corpuscles (nerves around hair follicles): When hair moves, the skin feels it. This evolutionary development provides additional awareness for wild animals. When people are nervous or scared, their skin develops goosebumps, which elevates the hair on the skin, which in turn becomes sensitive to the touch or the movement of air. When people report that they "sense it with my skin," they are referring to these nerves.

In addition to these sensory nerves, the skin also has motor nerves that move hair, constrict and relax blood vessels, and control sweat glands. They are the nerves responsible for blushing, goosebumps, shivering, and more.

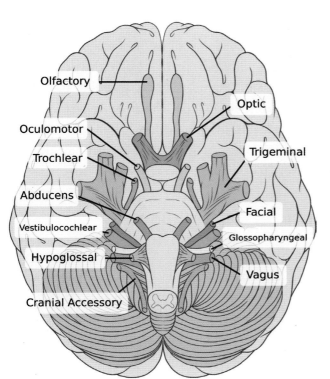

Figure 2.6.
The cranial nerves.
Illustration by Patrick J. Lynch, medical illustrator, and C. Carl Jaffe, M.D., cardiologist.

Every tissue in the body, including the skin, needs the electrical stimulation that is provided by the nerves. The skin has evolved through an abundance of nerve stimulation from the time the first humans experienced life in all its multisensorial richness. Today, when human skin is mostly covered by cloth, people spend most of their time in protected and conditioned environments; in addition, touching has become increasingly uncommon in many cultures so many people experience sensory starvation, where their skin does not receive the nerve stimulation it requires. Children and young adults typically have more movement, hugs, and physical contact with caregivers and one another. As people get older and embark on their individual journeys, however, they start starving their skin's nervous system of touch, thereby decreasing the number of nerve impulses going to the skin's cells. This too contributes to slower skin renewal and faster aging.

As well, negative emotions and stress increase muscle tension, which leads to wrinkling and causes the accumulation of inflammation-triggering neurochemicals that can wreak havoc on the skin's metabolism. Nowadays a common solution for dealing with wrinkles resulting from excessive muscle tension involves injections of botulinum toxin, which temporarily blocks nerve impulses in the areas most prone to wrinkles, such as the forehead and around the eyes and mouth. This may help smooth out wrinkles, but disrupts the flow of electricity through the skin. In contrast, the Taoist approach is based on awakening the skin's nerves and satiating sensory hunger while creating a deep relaxation response that favors regeneration and renewal.

THE SKIN'S CIRCULATION

The blood vessels that run through the skin are what brings energy to skin cells and tissues. They deliver nutrients and oxygen, which are used to produce energy. In the bottommost fatty layer as well as deep in the dermis there lie large- and medium-size blood vessels. These branch into smaller and smaller blood vessels, the capillaries. In the upper layer of the dermis, arterial capillaries form many tiny loops that become smaller and smaller until they change into venules and start forming

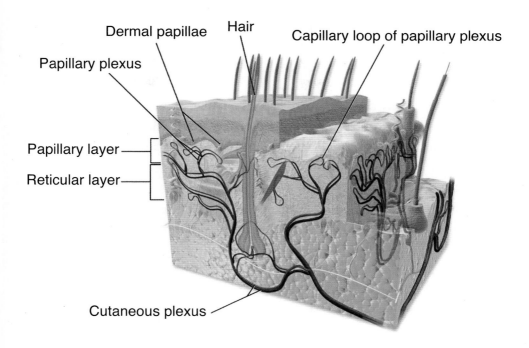

Figure 2.7. The blood vessels of the skin. Young, healthy skin has a rosy glow
that is created by blood flowing through the blood vessels.
Illustration by Blausen.com staff (2014),
"Medical Gallery of Blausen Medical 2014," CC 3.0.

bigger and bigger loops, returning deoxygenated blood to larger vessels. In young skin, arterial capillaries in the upper dermis form a dense layer of capillary loops. In one square millimeter of skin on the face, there could be up to 150 capillary loops.

When light penetrates the epidermis, the outermost layer of the skin, and reflects this dense pillow of blood vessels, it creates that celebrated rosy glow of youth. With age and especially stress, tiny capillaries start dying out. To compensate for this loss of the capillary network, larger blood vessels become larger. They form spiderlike structures, which lead to red spots on the cheeks and chin, a red nose, and visible enlarged veins under the skin. Taoist methods stimulate healthy circulation to restore oxygen and nutrient flow to the skin.

The skin's circulatory system is not only about blood; it also includes the lymphatic system, a network of channels lined with a single layer of flattened endothelial cells. These are the same cells that comprise the lining of the capillaries, but are more loosely connected. Lymph vessels detox the skin and replenish it with moisture. It is extremely important for the skin to have good lymph flow because without it skin cells will drown in waste, as no cleansers or soaps can remove accumulated toxic debris that suffocates skin cells. Tiny lymphatic vessels are like little streams that flow into larger vessels, carrying their waste-loaded fluids into the lymph nodes. Nobody really knows exactly what happens inside the lymph nodes, for they are not easy to study. But it is clear that the outflowing lymph is somehow detoxed and regenerated before it returns back to the lymph vessels. Each lymph node has a tough outer shell and soft lobes through which lymph slowly flows. These lobes are full of white blood cells, called *lymphocytes,* which kill bacteria and neutralize anything foreign.

To help the skin enjoy a cleaner and more vibrant inner environment it is essential that lymph moves through the skin and the rest of the body. The lymphatic vessels start in the mid-dermis and go deeper. There are no lymphatic vessels in the epidermis. Lymph moves throughout the body with stretching, movement, and the tensing and relaxing of tissues. With age, lymphatic vessels become fewer, which makes waste removal more difficult and less effective. It is frequently the case that as people age, they also start moving less. Even those who walk regularly or garden do not provide their skin's lymphatic system with sufficient stretching and vibration. This creates a toxic environment in the skin and blocks its renewal and regeneration.

Many massage practitioners and estheticians offer lymphatic drainage, which is a special massage technique to move lymph through the body. In the Taoist method, blood circulation and lymph flow, as well as skin cell renewal, are stimulated by using bamboo hitters that create deep-tissue vibration, a practice we shall discuss later in chapter 6.

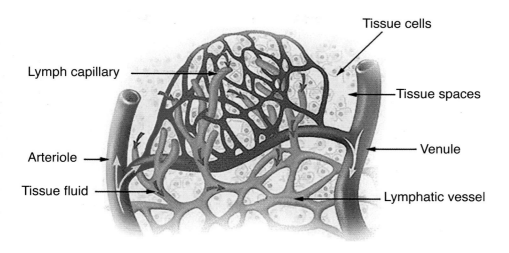

Figure 2.8. Lymphatic vessels in the skin remove waste
and provide hydration.

THE BREATH OF LIFE

Taoist sages believe that the body's life force is generated in the physical organs. Like the way fire burns to become light and heat or the way water, when boiling, becomes steam, so the human body has a burning mechanism in every cell that generates the electricity that is our life force.

In the 1770s French scientists Antoine Lavoisier and Pierre-Simon Laplace conducted an experiment in which they placed a guinea pig in a large sealed container immersed in a larger container filled with ice. The guinea pig was given enough food and water to survive. After ten hours, the animal's body heat melted thirteen ounces of ice in the outer container. Then they measured what at that time they called "fixed air," the substance the guinea pig breathed out while in confinement. Today we know that that what they termed "fixed air" was carbon dioxide, CO_2. Then the scientists measured how much coal they needed to burn to melt the same amount of ice and how much "fixed air" the burning process produced. The amount of CO_2 was almost identical. Now we know that the guinea pig's body, just like the human body, uses carbon from food and oxygen from air to produce CO_2. The process of burning coal similarly combines oxygen from the air with carbon from coal to produce CO_2. The guinea pig was "burning" carbon inside its cells to warm up its body and melt the ice. This was the first time that scientists demonstrated that an animal's body produces heat through a combustion process in which carbon, in the presence of oxygen, burns and releases CO_2. In an animal body (including humans) this process occurs slowly, in many complex steps that involve enzymes that regulate combustion. The nature of the process is the same as the way carbon from food is "burned" with oxygen so that CO_2 is released. Taoists teach that matter and energy are transformed into each other, exist within each other, and support each other. This concept is represented in the Tai Chi symbol of the interconnected yin and yang symbols. The Tai Chi symbol represents movement created by the interaction of opposites. Within yin there is always yang, and within yang there is always yin. They are not separate and they constitute a whole.

Our cells needs oxygen to make energy. The air we breathe enters the body through the lungs, which contain over 600 million air sacks, called *alveoli,* wrapped in blood vessels. If all the alveoli were stretched out to form a flat surface they would cover a tennis court—quite an impressive breathing surface! Because the lungs are not directly connected to other organs, including the skin, we need blood to deliver oxygen to the tissues and cells of the lungs and all the other organs. Like the lungs and all the other organs, the skin also absorbs oxygen and releases CO_2.

We can increase the amount of air we take in with every breath by opening our shoulders, relaxing our chest, and taking a deep breath by means of the abdominal and diaphragm muscles. How deeply those muscles move with each inhalation and exhalation determines how much air we take in. Modern life often forces us to spend most of our days crunched over a computer, which compresses the diaphragm and abdomen. Stress and anxiety further impede breathing, causing it to be shallow, and tight or layered clothing can sometimes interfere with the skin's ability to breathe. When breathing is insufficient, the tissues start accumulating CO_2, which creates a toxic and acidic environment. This leads to grayish, dull, sallow-looking skin as well as mysterious rashes and body aches. Even though there are cosmetic products and procedures that claim to improve the skin's oxygenation, in reality nothing can replace free, unrestricted, full-bodied breathing. (See directions for skin breathing on p. 82 and abdominal breathing on p. 218.)

Oxygen alone is not enough to produce the energy that will replenish the skin. Energy production requires fuel, which for the body comes in the form of food. Like oxygen that comes from the air we breathe, food doesn't just migrate from the digestive tract to the skin. The heart has to pump blood through the entire digestive tract, through the lungs, with their 600 million alveoli, and then to every skin cell, as well as to the rest of the body. The heart is approximately the size of a human fist, and yet it has to pump blood through an average of 100,000 miles of blood vessels. That's a lot of distance for blood cells to travel in order to carry oxygen and nutrients, and it's a lot of work for one human heart to pump blood through every vessel. When people get older, and especially if they are sedentary, some areas of the body will start receiving less blood. Stress and anxiety lead to constriction of the small blood vessels in the skin, further depriving it of fresh blood and therefore energy. Taoist Beauty Chi Kung practices focus on relaxation, breathwork, and mindful movement to help the skin as well as every organ in the body breathe with more ease in order to make more energy and thus create more radiance and beauty.

Five Rules of Beauty Chi Kung

   1. **Beautiful and radiant skin requires that we recharge the body's biobatteries.** In the West, our approach to productivity is deeply flawed because we are encouraged—even rewarded— to work ceaselessly, which makes stress and overwhelm a way of life. Chi Kung is a holistic remedy for stress. Instead of pushing the body to exhaustion, a Chi Kung practitioner takes great care to ensure that all the body's batteries are fully charged so that the essential needs of the body, and therefore the skin, are taken care of.

2. **Beauty is created by the breath of life.** Deep breathing and relaxation ensure energy production. No breath, no life. It is important to breathe well and deeply to create energy. A daily breathing meditation is the foundation of Beauty Chi Kung. In addition, one of the most effective ways to increase skin oxygenation and energy production is through Chi Kung Skin Breathing, a technique described in chapter 5.

3. **Beautiful skin means good circulation.** Relaxation and movement help move the blood through the body, ensuring that oxygen and nutrients are delivered to the cells. Chi Kung includes relaxation and stress-reducing exercises as well as gentle, mindful movements and self-massage.

4. **Healthy, glowing skin requires that we release adequate amounts of CO_2.** Ideally, CO_2 is removed from the tissues by blood cells and then released through the lungs. When breathing is shallow and the circulation is blocked, CO_2 is not going to magically disappear. It will be reabsorbed into the tissues, creating an unhealthy, toxic environment. When people hold back their negative emotions or are under stress, they do not breathe deeply and their skin consequently accumulates CO_2, creating a hypoxia state, which leads to an aged, dull complexion.

5. **Regeneration requires reducing stress and increasing the relaxation response.** When the body goes into a state of stress, the skin's surface capillaries constrict to prevent blood loss in case of wounding. If the stress is only brief, the skin can be supplied with its needs even if the breathing is shallow. If stress is chronic, however, the skin may not be getting enough of the oxygen it needs.

Thanks to Western science we have discovered much about human anatomy, biochemistry, and physiology that was not known to the ancient masters. However, this knowledge alone does not create beautiful skin. To develop one's inner beauty and outer radiance it is important to start taking action and commit to working holistically with the body, mind, and spirit.

In the East, the idea of doing inner work runs deep. For thousands of years, masters in India, China, Japan, and other Asian countries have understood the value of focused inner work to restructure one's energy. The great thing about the Taoist method is that all that's needed is a willingness to create time for practice and disciplined work. Without practice there is no transformation. Many people spend a lot of money on expensive retreats, workshops, and classes. Then they come home to the same old routine and wonder why nothing changes. The Taoist approach basically doesn't cost money. There is no need to buy expensive supplements, skin-care products, or exercise equipment.

Taoist masters teach that to make energy you need energy, just like making money requires investing money. Happiness, health, and beauty are treasures that require an investment of time and energy. It's important to put your "money"—i.e., your energy—in your body's "energy bank account," because otherwise you will have to deal with the consequences of years of self-neglect, which will be harder and harder to pay off as the years go by. Taoist practices create a stable stream of energy "income" into your energy bank account. In time, these practices become easy and enjoyable and yield great rewards.

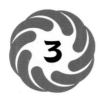

The Yin and Yang of Skin Renewal

Central to Taoist teachings is the concept of yin and yang, which can be explained as the balance of opposing forces that creates movement both in nature and in the human body. According to Taoist philosophy, there is no need to fight negative energy. This would only create imbalance. Whenever there is an excess of negative or even positive energy, it creates problems. Therefore it is important to understand that balance means finding equilibrium while in motion, similar to how a tightrope walker does not stand still, but walks by swaying to the left and to the right, adjusting and accommodating their body to constant change. The goal is not to be positive all the time, but to keep returning to balance. A momentary imbalance is needed to trigger motion, but then it is important to return to balance. Generally, yang is an expanding, hot, light, dry, active, doing, masculine energy, while yin is a gathering of cold, dense, heavy, dark, still, feminine energy. Men and women have both yin and yang energies. This idea of yin and yang balance is important when it comes to understanding how to keep the skin glowing and radiant.

There are many reasons why skin renewal slows down with age, but the two biggest ones are toxic inflammatory conditions and reduced blood flow due to impaired circulation. Skin beauty depends on the well-being of all the organs. If the lungs are not working properly, the skin will have less oxygen to make energy and it will consequently accumulate CO_2, which creates a toxic, acidic inner environment, which in turn impedes skin regeneration. With less oxygen available, the skin experiences hypoxic conditions that increase the production of free radicals that accelerate aging by damaging skin proteins, thereby creating wrinkles. If the liver is not working properly, the toxic byproducts of the body's metabolism will poison the skin and interfere with its renewal. If the kidneys aren't working properly, the skin will have to excrete more toxins, which will create a dull and aged-looking complexion. Kidney problems can also lead to water retention in the skin, swelling, and stagnation. If the heart is not working properly, the skin will not receive enough blood to make energy. If the skin's blood vessels are blocked or damaged, skin regeneration will be impaired. And if the digestive system does not supply the body with quality nutrients, the skin will not have energy and sufficient building blocks for renewal.

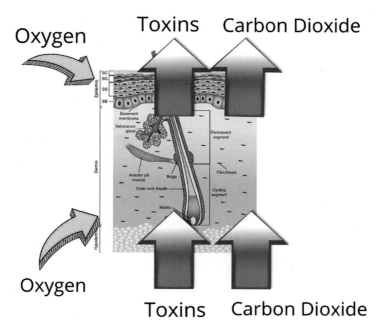

Figure 3.1. The skin helps absorb oxygen and removes CO_2 and toxins. When organs do not work well, the skin will start drowning in toxins.

Even though many cosmetic products and procedures promise to detox the skin, improve its circulation, and help it breathe, they will not work unless all the organs are working in balance and doing their jobs. There are many pharmaceutical drugs that are used to treat diseases of the internal organs. This is the Western approach, which has certain merits; however, these drugs also increase the toxic burden in the body, which is to say in the skin. Taoists believe that prevention is golden, so they have developed powerful practices for keeping the body healthy by balancing energy and ensuring good circulation, breathing, and optimal cleansing of the body.

THE NEGATIVE EFFECTS OF FLIGHT-OR-FLIGHT

The biggest factor that negatively influences skin in Western countries is stress and overwhelm. When the body is at peace (more yin), the capillaries are open and the skin feels warm and has a beautiful soft glow. Stress, on the other hand, activates the fight, flight, or freeze response. This inborn, ancient response helped our prehistoric forebears, who faced innumerable threats to their physical survival, escape danger.

When the fight-or-flight response is activated, the brain releases stress hormones such as corticotrophin-releasing hormone, glucocorticoids, and epinephrine, while the adrenal glands release adrenaline and cortisol. These hormones help an organism adapt to stress; however they also trigger a number of physiological responses that affect the skin's well-being. Because the skin faces the outer environment, it serves as a protective barrier and interface that is involved in detecting the first signs of danger through its sensitive receptors. It then responds to that stress physiologically. To have a better chance of survival, the body narrows the capillaries in the skin so they do not bleed much in case of an injury. While this is happening, more blood is directed to the arms and legs to enable the big muscles to work their best—enabling the "flight" part of the response. Meanwhile, the body releases energy from its reserves to ensure that every possible thing is being done to stay alive.

Humans have the same physiological reactions that our prehistoric and animal ancestors had, only now we rarely if ever have to run away from a lion or a bear. In place of those threats we have daily news, social media, workplace worries, and family conflicts. Since the skin has no eyes of its own, all visual information has to come to the skin through the brain, where it then turns into a mental image. It is this mental image that triggers the fight-or-flight response. The skin really cannot distinguish whether something is being received through the eyes and then turned into a mental image in the brain, or whether it started out as a thought. It only knows that the body is under attack.

When you see an actual snake, the brain creates a mental picture of a snake, which triggers a stress response. But a mental image of a snake can also trigger a stress response, as in what happens when you mistake a rope for a snake.

In the distant past, our human ancestors, like most animals, spent most of their time at peace. When a predator or any other danger appeared, they would spring into action and either fight or run away. When someone is stressed-out (a yang condition), the tiny capillaries in their skin become constricted and the blood cannot flow freely. If the stress lasts for just a short time it's not an issue. However, in modern life, stresses never seem to go away. Every day there is a new challenge, and if there is not enough stress in a person's life the media is always ready to provide some. Modern professionals take great pride in their ability to perform under pressure, and they constantly push themselves to exhaustion; however, the human body still obeys the same rules it did in the distant past. The human brain may be fooled into thinking that daily stress is normal and even exhilarating, but the body will activate the same fight-or-flight response it has been activating since the dawn of time. When stress becomes chronic and there is no peace or rest, the body starts producing more and more cortisol, which weakens the immune system and triggers inflammation. Chronic stress and anxiety interfere with breathing, which becomes shallow, impairs digestion, disrupts sleep, and further prevents the body from getting much-needed rest. Also, chronic worry and unhappiness create habitual muscle tension in the facial muscles, which leads to wrinkling. Yes, injections of botulinum toxin can help smooth those wrinkles temporarily, but once the results of the injection fade, the tension is back.

The longer the body maintains tension, the more the skin suffers, and it will develop a dull, pale, grayish, lifeless appearance due to impaired renewal function and the accumulation of CO_2 and other metabolic wastes. Gradually the corners of the mouth go down and the whole face sags and starts looking disgruntled. Another danger of stress is the increase of inflammation it brings, and this can evolve into a chronic state. Scientists have discovered that chronic low-grade inflammation caused by stress is the major accelerator of aging in all tissues, including the skin. Researchers have coined the term *inflamm-aging* to describe this.[1] Stress has been shown to aggravate the symptoms of atopic dermatitis, acne, psoriasis, and skin allergies. And any invasive cosmetic procedures can result in complications and a longer recovery time if the person is chronically stressed.

To understand what stress does to the skin, we can imagine a village where all its residents are living in peace. They work hard every day to have enough food to feel safe and secure, and they have enough time to rest, repair their homes, produce art, dance, laugh, and make love. Similarly, the skin repairs and regenerates when the mind and body are at rest. The skin needs relaxed muscles and capillaries, enough oxygen, and a prompt release of CO_2 to remain radiant and beautiful. When a person is chronically stressed there is no time to rest, dance, make love, or repair your home. All the body's reserves are basically at war. That is why the skin cannot adequately repair and renew when the mind and body are constantly on high alert and the tissues are flooded with inflammatory molecules.

THE IMPORTANCE OF STILLNESS
AND INNER FOCUS

Taoists have emphasized the importance of rest and relaxation for thousands of years, but it took an epidemic of stress in modern times before Western science finally started researching the effects of constant unhappiness and overwhelm. In the human body there are two nervous systems, the sympathetic and the parasympathetic.

- The **sympathetic nervous system** is considered a yang system because it activates when we are active, busy, expanding, and exploring. It is also active when the body is in danger or has to deal with a challenge.
- The **parasympathetic nervous system** is considered a yin system because it activates when the body is resting, digesting food, relaxing, repairing, and regenerating. The sympathetic and parasympathetic nervous systems complement each other just like yin and yang.

The body needs both systems to be flowing, stimulated, and moving toward a brighter future, since life without any stress at all would be dull and boring. Overcoming challenges and feeling fear, anger, excitement, and frustration add spice to life and fill it with a sense of adventure. A good boost of adrenaline feels good sometimes. The skin needs the ebb and flow of emotions to stimulate its circulation. Excitement makes the blood flow faster, and fear momentarily constricts the capillaries so that when they open again they can fill with fresh blood.

On the other hand, constant stress and overwhelm can become a way of life. Stress can be okay when the body is young because it has abundant energy reserves. But as the body ages, it cannot withstand the rigors of chronic stress because it cannot generate enough energy to repair the damage it has caused. All the organs are vital, and they receive less energy when the whole body is exhausted. And of all the organs, the skin is most likely to become energy-depleted because such a big surface area must regenerate. If energy is never replenished as when stress and overwhelm is constant, the skin will accumulate damage and develop blemishes, discoloration, inflammation, and a dull, gray appearance. And of course the rest of the body will also suffer from any number of conditions caused by the accumulation of metabolic wastes.

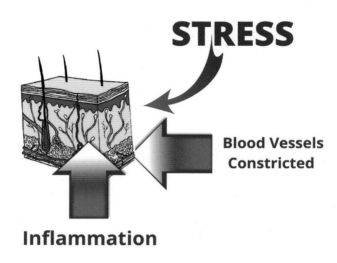

Figure 3.2. Stress triggers the fight-or-flight response, which sends more blood to the big muscles in the arms and legs while constricting the skin's blood vessels, leading to inflammation.

TEACHING THE BODY TO REST AND RELAX

When there is an abundant flow of golden energy, the skin will appear clear and radiant. In contrast, when energy is depleted as a result of stress, the skin will attempt to save the day by agreeing to make more of its resources available to the rest of the body so it can address the even more pressing needs of the other organs. That is why it's essential to open the body to the flow of energy, or chi. Mindful relaxation is the very foundation of Beauty Chi Kung. If the body is not relaxed and open to the flow of chi, no cosmetics, cosmetic procedures, or nutritional wonders will work, because what the body really needs is energy. Rest and relaxation doesn't mean you must quit your high-paying job in order to move to a cave in the mountains. But it does mean reclaiming the lost art of stillness and inner focus. Children and animals know how to relax naturally and do not need lessons in relaxation. Nowadays, however, as people mature, they learn to adapt to constant stress and forget how to let it go.

Throughout the ages, spiritual masters have emphasized the importance of a quiet mind and a relaxed, peaceful body on the path to enlightenment. The same qualities are needed to maintain the skin's radiance, health, and beauty. Stress, worry, and toxic and negative emotions might go along with accomplishing more than is humanly possible, but they eventually deplete the life force, increase inflammation, and destroy the skin's health and beauty. A human body is not designed to live in stress indefinitely. Someone who forgets how to feel safe and relaxed may end up battling a host of health problems, including inflammation, suppressed immunity and greater susceptibility to viruses and bacterial infections, high blood pressure, disruptions in glucose metabolism, impaired digestion, low sexual drive, and more.

Relaxation is a skill that can be mastered. No matter how stressful the events in the outside world are, it is crucially important that we relax. Just a few minutes of relaxation can give the skin that much-needed break to replenish and regenerate its resources. Note that watching TV or drinking alcohol is *not* relaxation. TV may distract the mind, which welcomes a shift in activity, but the body still needs to expend energy to process the information from the screen, just as it will need energy to detox from alcohol and repair any damage caused by excessive consumption. And these days, watching the news is probably the worst stressor of all. To relax truly, it is important to really communicate to the body that it is safe, at least in the moment.

In the next chapter we will introduce the Inner Smile meditation, a Taoist mindful relaxation practice that is used to destress the body, create a peaceful, grounded state of mind, and restore the flow of chi in the organs.

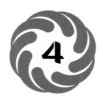

The Five Elements and Inner Smile for Radiant Skin

Over five thousand years ago, Taoist masters discovered three powerful medicines: breathing, smiling, and moving. Master Mantak Chia's Taoist teacher, White Cloud Hermit, often said, "If you take care of the five major organs, you take care of hundreds and thousands of problems. If you do not take care of the five major organs, you will have to deal with hundreds and thousands of problems. And then you have to take hundreds and thousands of medicines." Ancient Taoists viewed sickness and problems in the organs as being like blocks of ice. Smiling is a sunshine that melts ice and turns it first into water, and then into steam. When ice is melted by smiling sunshine, life, light, and healing become possible.

The skin, as we know, has its own renewal, regeneration, and rejuvenation power. Like the other organs it too needs love and healing vibrations to activate these powers. Relaxing and smiling loving energy into one's body helps the skin release endorphins, which opens capillary blood flow and accelerates healing. It also helps produce oxytocin, the love and bonding hormone that has been shown to reduce overall inflammation, encourage regeneration, release muscle tension, reduce cortisol, lower the inflammatory response, and restore youthful radiance and glow to the skin. Have you noticed that when people are in love their faces look younger and more radiant? It's because of the chemical symphony of love illuminating the skin from within.

The Inner Smile is the foundational practice of Taoist Chi Kung. It involves generating love toward yourself and toward your entire body. Taoists believe that the Inner Smile connects us to universal unconditional love. It establishes good communication between all the inner organs and the outermost organ, the skin. Taoists believe that if people learn to smile at their problems, they would have a much better chance at finding solutions. Many emotional problems can be resolved by bringing the problem state into a more resourceful and powerful inner state. According to the Tao, it is possible to heal your own body through a smiling meditation practice that follows a specific pattern discovered thousands of years ago called the *five elements creating cycle*. It's just as effective, if not more so, than repeating mantras or trying to empty your mind, as with other meditative techniques, and offers additional benefits of restoring flow of chi in the organs, de-stressing the body, and creating a beautiful healthy glow in one's skin.

THE FIVE ELEMENTS CREATING CYCLE

The five elements are fire, earth, metal, water, and wood. They are connected in a harmonious creative cycle: fire produces ashes to create more earth; earth grows and creates more metal; metal grows and attracts more water; water grows and creates more wood; and wood grows and creates more fire. This sequence is easy to remember and it communicates to the unconscious mind the idea of harmony and co-creation as an interconnected whole. This is exactly what is needed to help the skin replenish and become more radiant. Since the human body possesses an innate ability to return to balance and heal itself, communicating the idea of harmonious creative teamwork among all the systems of the body helps the body return to balance. Each element has its own energy, which is represented visually as a color, kinesthetically as a set of feelings, and symbolically as a season and a sacred animal. Every organ

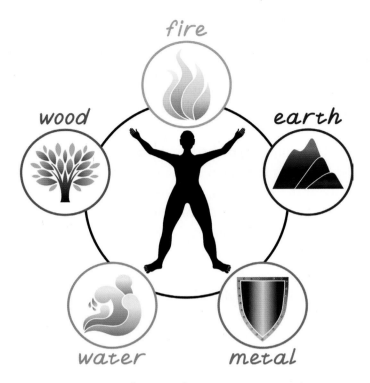

Figure 4.1 The Five Elements Creating Cycle

is linked to an element. This method allows for an easy sorting of the emotions in the body according to the organs and helps us connect to the organs nonverbally.

- In the Taoist tradition, the heart and small intestine are con- nected to the **fire** element and the color **red.** Fire represents expanding and radiating energy, which, when unbalanced, can turn into destructive burning energy. It is connected to **summer,** with its hot, radiant days and abundant growth.
- The spleen, pancreas, and stomach are linked to the **earth** element and the color **yellow.** Earth energy is serene, calming, and nourish- ing, but it can become shaky and uncertain when unbalanced. It is connected to **late summer** (early autumn), with its warm, golden glow of colorful foliage and plentiful bounty in the fields.

- The lungs and large intestine are connected to the **metal** element (lungs are also connected to the skin since the skin is considered the "third lung") and the color **white.** Metal energy is solidifying and clear, and can turn into cutting and heavy energy when unbalanced. It is connected to **fall,** with its colder days and decreased activity.
- The kidneys and bladder are connected to the **water** element and the color **blue.** Water is cooling, flowing, calming, and resilient,

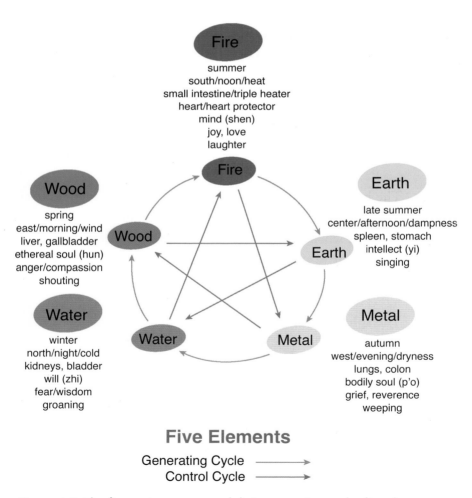

Figure 4.2. The five major organs and their connection to the five elements.

and can be freezing and drowning when unbalanced. Water's season is **winter,** with its freezing landscapes and stillness.

- The liver and gallbladder are associated with the **wood** element and the color **green.** Wood is warm, moist, generous, rich, and can take over and grow in all directions when unbalanced. It is connected to **spring,** with its bold, new growth and buds bursting with life force.

The change of seasons has traditionally been significant for humans, since season symbolism speaks powerfully to the unconscious mind. The Inner Smile involves smiling into each organ and meditating on its corresponding element and the energies associated with it. This practice balances the energy of the organ involved and clears it of negative energy. At first it takes some time to remember the sequence and the colors, but with repeated practice this exercise is quite easy and enjoyable.

When you have memorized the colors and the sequence, you can start exploring how the organs work with chi.

- The **heart** and **small intestine** have the positive energies of the fire element, which are love, joy, and happiness, and the negative energies, which are hatred, cruelty, judgment, impatience, and rage. Negative energies of the fire element can make the skin hot, red, tense, and inflamed. Positive emotions of the fire element increase skin radiance and beauty.
- The **spleen, pancreas,** and **stomach** have the positive energies of the earth element, which are trust, faith, and confidence; the negative energies are mistrust, anxiety, worry, and self-doubt. Negative energies of the earth element can make the skin tense, dull, withdrawn, ashen, and gray, while faith and confidence, which are positive energies of the earth element, increase radiance and beauty.
- The **lungs** and **large intestine** have the positive energies of the metal element, which are courage and righteousness. The negative energies of the lungs and large intestine are grief, depression,

and sadness. They draw the life out of the skin, making it appear grayish, lifeless, and pale. Grief can prematurely age the skin and turn hair gray. Courage and righteousness, which are positive energies of the metal element, help create a more uplifted and glowing complexion.

- The **kidneys** and **bladder** have the positive energies of the water element, which are calmness, tranquility, and gentleness. The negative energies are fear and stress, which can make the skin tense, constrict its capillaries, and diminish its renewal and radiance. When the skin radiates these qualities it looks younger and more attractive and has a calming effect on other people.

- The **liver** and **gallbladder** have the positive energy of the wood element, which are generosity and kindness. The negative energies are greed, jealousy, and anger. They increase skin tension, block its radiance, and accelerate wrinkles. Kindness and generosity impart a more relaxed and radiant expression.

THE POWER OF A TRUE SMILE

The Inner Smile is the Taoist mindful relaxation meditation. It may initially take some time to learn, but once mastered it can be done in just a few minutes.

First, it is very important to learn *how* to smile. In the Tao, a smile is not used to hide one's true feelings, but instead becomes a powerful healing tool. To be a healing tool, a smile has to be a genuine smile of pure, unconditional love that blossoms from the heart and illuminates one's whole being. The miracle of a true, genuine, loving smile cannot be underestimated. In the Tao, a constant loving smile at oneself—an inward smile—is the foundation for all our energy work.

Taoist masters hold that the body is a temple and every organ a shrine that deserves our attention and reverence. In every religion there are images that the people who practice that religion hold in their minds. Taoists suggest we start doing the same thing with our internal organs. Instead of prayers and mantras, Taoists use a simple, loving smile. When you smile a genuinely loving smile, it's like smiling a sunshine that can melt ice and awaken your inner healing light. The Inner Smile is the secret door that can lead you to truly love yourself. It sends good images and good energy throughout the body. It floods the body with soothing endorphins and the happy chemicals of serotonin, dopamine, and oxytocin. It calms and relaxes the organs and stimulates digestion, absorption, and the removal of wastes. It activates healing and regeneration. It's our best medicine, and it's absolutely free!

Today we have the multibillion-dollar entertainment industry and a multibillion-dollar food industry whose products advertisers claim can create happy feelings. If that's the case, why are so many people still unhappy when they finish watching a movie or eating that yummy cake? The Inner Smile, when practiced daily, creates natural feelings of joy and happiness, which makes the skin glow beautifully. It gives the body a break from constant stress so that the skin can repair itself and get back into balance.

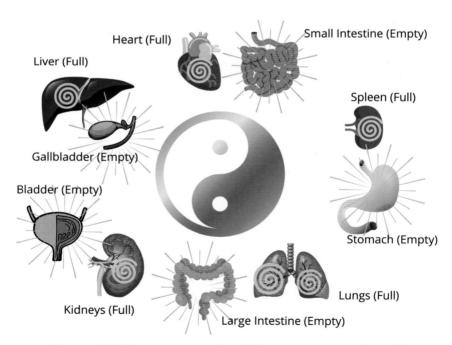

Figure 4.3. Yin organs store chi, while yang organs radiate chi.
Yang organs are empty and yin organs are full.

Before you begin this practice, make sure you know the locations and shapes of the five major organs so you can easily visualize them. The Inner Smile, which follows the Five Elements Creating Cycle as illustrated in figure 4.1 (p. 64), helps balance the negative and positive energies of each organ. When the shapes and locations of the organs as well as their corresponding colors, elements, and energies are memorized, it's easy to amplify their vibrant and radiant energy and release any dark, cloudy, murky, muddy energy.

WHEN TO PRACTICE THE INNER SMILE

As our foundational practice, the Inner Smile has to be done daily. Every day, gravity and negative emotions pull the skin downward and fill it with toxins, so it is very important to do something to counteract these influences. Make sure you always smile inwardly when you work with your own body. The Inner Smile is best done in the morning. Once you develop the habit of smiling into your own body with unconditional love, you no longer have to deal with grumpiness and sluggishness in the morning. Some people find that once they've mastered the Inner Smile and it becomes a habit, they no longer need their morning coffee!

The Inner Smile helps the facial muscles stay uplifted and energized, which counteracts gravity and prevents the skin from sagging. It also saturates the skin with endorphins, which relax the tiny capillaries within the skin, filling it with a beautiful, healthy glow and helping the skin cells make more chi. It stimulates the production of oxytocin, which reduces inflammation and helps establish better social connections. It also elevates serotonin, which helps breathing and digestion, which in turn helps make more chi. Finally, it creates more dopamine, which is associated with a sense of accomplishment and can make a person feel more confident and beautiful.

There are dozens of other molecular messengers and neurotransmitters that are activated by the Inner Smile, so smiling at your organs in the morning can be compared to drinking a multifunctional health elixir that uplifts, energizes, beautifies, boosts confidence, and reduces stress.

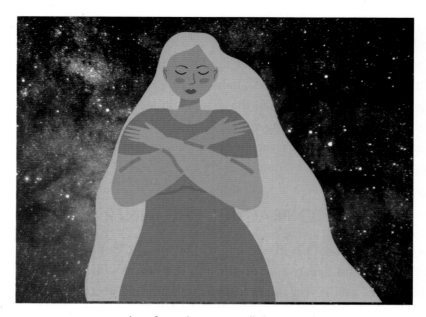

Figure 4.4. Smiling from the crown all the way down creates a
waterfall of unconditional love.

Even though a quick waterfall-style Inner Smile as described below is
very beneficial, it is important to also go through the full Five Elements
Creating Cycle as often as possible. This cycle follows the natural pro-
gression of the five elements: **fire** (red, heart, small intestine) burns and
creates ashes to build **earth** (yellow, spleen, pancreas, stomach), which
gives birth to **metal** (white, lungs, large intestine), which attracts **water**
(blue, kidneys and bladder), which grows **wood** (green, liver and gallbladder), which can be burned to create more fire and thus begin the
cycle all over again. It unites all the organs into one chi flow, establishing harmony and cooperation and saturating them with happy chemicals
that balance digestion, absorption, and elimination. Depending on one's
time, the meditation can be shortened to focusing on just the colors and
the organs and saturating them with unconditional love, or it can go
deeper into the emotional energy associated with each element. The best
way to practice is to go through the cycle at least nine times per session.

Inner Smile Chi Kung

This simple practice can take anywhere from a few seconds to ten or fifteen minutes if you do the full cycle nine times. The simplest Inner Smile can be as easy as smiling from the crown down, imagining the smile like a waterfall nourishing every organ and every cell. This can be done while waiting for the traffic light to change or sitting in the waiting room of a doctor's office. If you have no time for any other practice, do the Inner Smile, and you will notice how having more energy and a more uplifted and happy body makes daily tasks much easier and more enjoyable.

1. Sit on the edge of a chair with your feet flat on the floor and your body relaxed. Put your hands on your lap. Notice if you are more comfortable with your palms up or down or one palm under the other. Close your eyes or just make them very heavy and relaxed. Now think about someone you love. It's best to select the feeling of unconditional love, such as toward your child or your grandchild, or an animal such as your dog or cat. You can also imagine a beautiful and serene place that stirs feelings of love.
2. Smile slightly by lifting the corners of your mouth.
3. Imagine unconditional love as a cloud of golden light.
4. Take a deep breath through your nose, inhaling the energy of the unconditional love as a cloud of golden light. As you inhale, simultaneously, roll your eyes up, look up into your brain and smile the golden light into your brain. Exhale and relax your eyes. Repeat a few times until you really feel it.
5. Return to smiling into the golden cloud of unconditional love in front of you
6. Next, inhale the smiling energy of love again, and as you exhale, smile into your eyes. Imagine your eyes and your mind shining loving sunshine. Think love, happiness, respect, and gratitude. You can repeat this step a few times until your eyes begin to feel loving, smiling sensations. The Tao teaches to think of golden rays of sunshine gently shining on a surface of water, creating a warm and nice feeling.

7. Next, become aware of your heart. Inhale, smiling loving energy, looking into your heart and smiling loving sunshine into your heart. Imagine your heart as a red rose that slowly opens its petals to fullness. Visualize a warm, loving fire growing in your heart. Visualize the energy of love, joy, and happiness as the warm red mist that spreads from your heart until it starts radiating through your skin.

8. Look down at your abdomen and smile into your small intestine. Invoke the feelings of joy, love, and happiness. Keep smiling golden sunshine.

9. Bring your attention to your spleen, pancreas, and stomach, and smile. Visualize moving the loving energy from the small intestine to your spleen, pancreas, and stomach. Imagine your spleen, pancreas, and stomach opening and growing as a yellow rose. Invoke the feelings of trust and confidence. Visualize trust, confidence, and faith as the yellow mist that grows and radiates through your skin. Imagine earth energy, which is stable, solid, and supportive. Visualize moving loving, smiling energy to the lungs.

10. Smile into your lungs. Imagine your lungs opening and growing as a white rose. Invoke the feeling of courage as metal energy, which is cool, dry, strong, open, and direct. Visualize courage in your lungs as the white mist that spreads and radiates through your skin. Next, visualize moving smiling, loving energy into your kidneys.

11. Smile into your kidneys. See your kidneys opening and growing like a blue rose. Invoke the feelings of calmness and tranquility as water energy, which is flowing, calm, and serene. Imagine calmness and serenity as the blue mist that grows, spreads, and radiates through your skin. Next, move smiling, loving energy to your liver.

12. Smile into your liver. Imagine your liver opening and growing like a green rose. Invoke the feelings of kindness, generosity, and wood energy, which is growing and expanding and giving life to fire. Let the energies of kindness and generosity spread and radiate through your skin as green mist.

13. Return to your heart and imagine adding more wood to the fire and watching its loving fire growing.

14. Repeat this Five Elements Creating Cycle nine times. With every round, your heart fire will grow and radiate, your earth energy will become stronger, your metal energy will grow, and your water will flow more abundantly to help your forest grow so you can create more and more love.

The Inner Smile is an instant face-lift that increases your glow and radiance, creates a more attractive and inviting aura, and helps you generate a positive impression as it boosts your confidence and self-esteem and makes you appear younger, healthier, and more vital. Many people have reported emerging from this practice feeling replenished and rejuvenated, their skin glowing and shining. Beauty, which flows freely when we're young and diminishes when we get older, can be replenished, restored, and regenerated from within through mindful inner practices such as this.

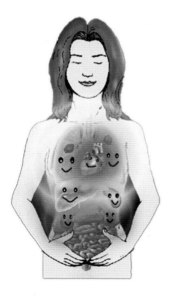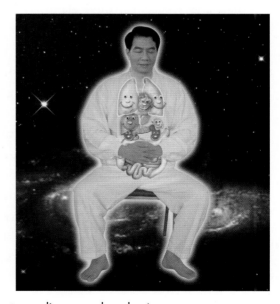

Figure 4.5. The Inner Smile creates radiance and a glowing presence.
It's the link to unconditional love.

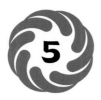

Breathing Life into Skin

The human body has over five million pores, some 20,000 located in the facial area alone. Since beauty standards favor smooth, flawless skin, many people whose skin has larger and more visible pores do their best to mask, cover, and tighten them. Skin pores are actually openings for hair and sebaceous (oily) glands, which produce a waxlike substance commonly known as skin oil.

For women, of course, facial hair, with the exception of hair growing on the head, eyebrow and eyelashes, is a nuisance, and is often removed by means of plucking, waxing, chemical depilatories, electrolysis, or laser hair removal. Hair on the rest of the body typically follows the same fate. In modern Western culture, both facial and body hair on women is unwanted. Since beauty standards call for velvety, nongreasy skin, skin oil is also considered a nuisance, and women whose skin produces more oil do their best to remove it. All in all, most women, if given a choice, would prefer not to have any pores at all and ideally have smooth, even skin. In this chapter, you will learn that skin pores, oil, and hair, regardless of their location, are biologically and energetically important features of the skin.

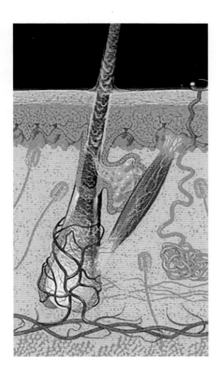

Figure 5.1. Skin oil gland and hair follicle structure.

BREATHING THROUGH YOUR PORES

Taoists believe that every pore is an opening for chi, and every hair can serve as an antenna that draws more chi into the skin. They developed a unique technology of skin breathing, which helps draw more chi into the body through every pore. Modern women can greatly benefit from this technology because it helps stimulate skin circulation and metabolism and awakens the stem cells located in the hair follicles.

It is important to notice that unless we are talking about frogs, skin breathing does not provide significant amounts of oxygen to the body. However skin breathing *is* vital for the skin. The very top layer of the skin, the epidermis, the layer that is visible to others, does not have its own blood vessels and has to receive all its oxygen from the air or from underlying tissues. It has been established that oxygen can dissolve in oily substances, so skin oil, especially skin oil located in the pores, is the perfect solution for binding and storing oxygen to supply the skin's needs. Ancient Taoists used to temporarily hold their breath to activate skin breathing and to create the conditions that allow the skin to draw more vital energy into the pores. As the ancient masters used to say, "When the real breath stops, the true breath begins." Many traditions have various breathing techniques for spiritual and physical advancement. In Vedic philosophy, breathing techniques are used to work with prana, which is the equivalent of chi and is believed to permeate all living and inanimate objects and everything in the universe. Those who practice yoga are likely familiar with some of these breathing techniques. What distinguishes the Taoist approach is that this particular skin breathing technique is simple, easy to learn, and does not require prolonged holding of the breath or years of practice. It can be used by anyone to activate the skin's energy, stimulate its breathing, and bring more energy to its stem cells.

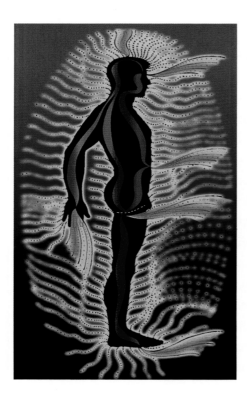

Figure 5.2. Skin breathing according to the Tao. Every pore is an opening for chi, and every hair can serve as an antenna to draw more chi into the skin.

SKIN ENERGY BREATHING

Taoists hold that in addition to chi produced in the body from food and oxygen, human beings can absorb chi from nature, other people, and even celestial bodies. These beliefs perhaps seem outlandish, but then again humans created modern technologies for the wireless transmission of electromagnetic energy when just a century ago Wi-Fi would have been considered magic. Now we can send complex messages and images to the opposite side of the world in a matter of seconds, and we get annoyed if the connection is too slow. If humans can create technology that enables wireless communication, it is quite possible that human neurology, which is very complex, already possesses the technology and wiring to receive, transmit, and transform energy. This energy can be used to replenish, recharge, and reenergize fading and lifeless skin.

Thousands of years ago, Taoists taught that the whole universe is filled with violet light, which has healing power, wisdom, and intelligence. They concluded that if the whole universe is filled with this wondrous light, then it is everywhere, including in the space around us. They maintained that we can absorb light through our skin, skull, and body energy centers.

According to Taoist wisdom, when a fetus in the womb cannot breathe oxygen through the lungs and has to receive oxygen and nutrition through the umbilical cord, they receive the universal wisdom light through their skin, skull, and body energy centers. After a baby is born and starts breathing air, he or she is still breathing the light (in Vedic tradition, as prana) until the baby grows older, starts thinking (and even overthinking), gets busy with life, and disconnects from the light.

Taoist skin breathing involves creating suction in the abdominal area, which in the Tao is called the Lower Tan Tien, and then using this suction to draw chi into the pores. Every hair can be an antenna extending out into the universe, drawing the universal healing light in. Even though this may seem farfetched, modern science is beginning to discover that the Taoist practice of skin breathing has some very real foundations.

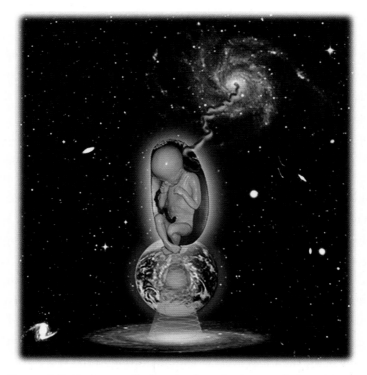

Figure 5.3. Taoists teach that the fetus in the womb breathes the high-vibrational violet light that permeates the universe.

Recently, biologist and molecular geneticist Johnjoe McFadden, at the University of Surrey, England, proposed the Consciousness Electromagnetic Information (Cemi) Field theory, which claims that "consciousness is that component of the brain's electromagnetic field that is downloaded to motor neurons and is thereby capable of communicating its informational content to the outside world."[1] Basically, what this means is that electromagnetic energy can be structured into electromagnetic clouds of structured energy that are conscious. Many scientists agree that one of the functions of the body's nervous system is to structure electromagnetic energy into these Cemi fields, similar to how modern computers structure electromagnetic energy into information. This supports the ancient Taoist idea that the energy of the mind is quite real and can be structured by the body-mind. It also explains why the skin can be noticeably illuminated by a bright idea, an inspiration, a passion, or love. If thoughts are made out of structured clouds of electromagnetic energy, then they quite possibly can create a shining radiance that can be easily observed on the faces of people in love. It seems the ancient Taoists were right, and our vast universe can generate consciousness too. Modern research has begun to move toward this conclusion. Just recently, astronomers discovered the existence of a cosmic web consisting of gigantic strings of gaseous matter and faint light that forms a web of interconnected, intergalactic energy filaments in deep space. These structures have a strange resemblance to structures found in the human brain, which is "composed by water (77–78 percent), lipids (10–12 percent), proteins (8 percent), carbohydrates (1 percent), soluble organic substances (2 percent), salt (1 percent); the Universe is made for a 73~ percent by Dark Energy (a scalar energy field of the empty space), for a 22.5 percent by Dark Matter, for 4.4 percent by ordinary baryonic matter and for less than 0.1 percent by photons and neutrinos."[2]

Recently, scientists have confirmed the existence of forms of non-chemical and nonneurological communications between cells.[3] In one

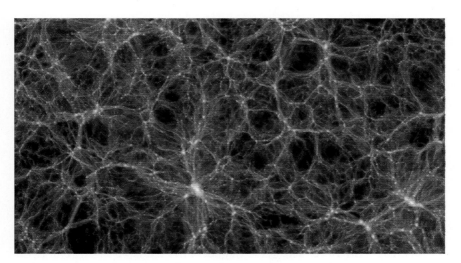

Figure 5.4. The cosmic "brain" discovered in space bears an uncany resemblance to the human brain.

experiment, cells were separated into two separate cell cultures; one culture was exposed to hydrogen peroxide (toxic for cells), which resulted in cellular damage and a 46 percent decrease in protein synthesis. It was confirmed that even though the cells in the other cell culture were not exposed to hydrogen peroxide and were not directly damaged, they nevertheless reduced their protein synthesis similar to the group of cells that were treated with hydrogen peroxide. This offers some proof that all the cells in the body communicate with one another through a biological version of Wi-Fi.

SKIN BREATHING ENLIVENS THE PORES

The Taoist method of skin breathing involves the pores and their function. What is visible on the surface as a skin pore is actually the opening of a very complex structure called the *pilosebaceous unit.* There is another kind of a skin pore that is so small it is not visible to the naked eye, which is the opening for the apocrine, or sweat glands; however these types of pores do not factor into skin breathing because they are so small.

To understand the structure of the pilosebaceous unit, one can imagine pressing a tiny needle into the skin that causes all the layers of the skin to press inward until they create an invagination, such that the layer of dead, cornified, flattened cells of the epidermis—what was on the outside surface—is now on the inside. As is true everywhere in the epidermis, the cells in the opening of a skin pore are constantly shedding and being replaced by new cells. At the same time, skin oil is being secreted from the same opening. This means that the skin cells shedding from the surface and skin oil can get mixed together in the pore. If the skin produces too much sebum, and if this sebum is too thick, or if the skin pore is clogged by cosmetics, or if skin cells are not shedding properly, or some combination of all of this, the skin pore will get clogged. This leads to enlargement of the sebaceous glands and the appearance of visible comedones, which are small bumps or blemishes. At first this results in whiteheads, but when the oily substance oxidizes and mixes with pigments, the result is blackheads. If the skin pores remain clogged, the sebaceous glands get backed up with sebum and become enlarged. Eventually the pore becomes bigger and more visible. There is a microorganism that lives in the oily glands because it loves skin oil; this is *Propionibacterium acne* (*P. acne*), which produces irritating and inflammation-inducing fatty acids that wreak havoc on the skin. Even though comedones and acne are considered a teenage problem, many people over forty still struggle with oily skin, clogged pores, and acne.

It has been demonstrated that those who struggle with adult acne are also predisposed to having more inflammation in the skin. Their skin is often sensitive, has more nerve endings than the average, and produces more inflammatory molecules, such as the neuropeptides IL-1 and TGF-beta. These molecules affect the oil glands, increasing their size, stimulating excessive sebum secretion, and disrupting cell exfoliation in the oil gland lining. As a result, the pore opening becomes plugged with a thick mixture of sebum and skin cells.

In the past it was believed that people who struggle with adult acne and skin oiliness have too much of the chemical dihydrotestosterone in their skin, which is an active form of the male sexual hormone testosterone. However it is now established that in addition to testosterone there are many other chemicals in the skin that can trigger excessive oil production and cause oil gland enlargement. Among these are human growth hormone (hGH), which explains teenage acne, as well as the other hormones associated with stress. So in many cases the combination of higher skin sensitivity along with stress may be the main reason the skin's oil glands get out of balance. Taoist skin breathing includes relaxation and mindfulness, which is proven to release stress and reduce inflammation in the body.

Another reason why Taoist skin breathing is so effective is because of the fact that electromagnetic energy in the human body moves with our conscious attention. The simple practice of bringing more attention to the skin's surface and enhancing this attention by "breathing" into the skin is enough to stimulate the nerves, increase circulation, and thereby affect cell renewal. It is very important to do this practice in a calm, relaxed, peaceful state of mind to encourage the formation of "happy chemicals" such as endorphins, oxytocin, and serotonin. Developing confidence in one's practice will add dopamine to the mix, which also helps increase the skin's radiance.

HOW TO BREATHE LIFE INTO THE SKIN

Ancient Taoist masters did not have our modern electronics, nevertheless they developed astonishing technologies that rely on the mind-body connection. Nowadays, energy can be generated and moved by the movement of the wind and water turbines; in the body, energy is generated and moved through the movement of the mind and the breath, as in the following exercise.

Skin-Breathing Chi Kung*

This powerful practice detoxes, stimulates, and activates skin and hair follicle cells while it replenishes the skin with chi. The practice takes some time to learn, but once mastered it can be done anywhere, anytime. It's a great practice to do outdoors in a beautiful natural setting so the skin can receive clean, natural chi. It can be combined with Iron Shirt Chi Kung, found in chapter 10 , or just done on its own. It also works well with Stem Cell Chi Kung using a bamboo hitter, described in chapter 6, a practice that activates the circulation and awakens stem cells as it detoxes and energizes the skin and its underlying tissues. All these practices assist in the absorption of biologically active components in cosmetic products as well as restoring chi to the skin.

It is important that you prepare your skin for Skin-Breathing Chi Kung. Remove all makeup and wash your face with warm water and a

---

*Skin and hair breathing are also described in Master Mantak Chia's book *Elixir Chi Kung.*

mild, pH-balanced skin cleanser. In some cases, using a mild exfoliating product may help open the skin's pores and prepare them to receive more chi. Most importantly, take time to relax and create a mental space for this practice. It's best to do it outdoors in a clean, natural environment, but if this isn't possible, imagine a peaceful nature scene before beginning the practice.

Note: This practice includes a brief period of holding your breath. Make sure this is done within a comfortable range. There should be no dizziness or any other discomfort.

1. Stand with your feet shoulder-width apart, toes pointed straight forward. Keep your shoulders relaxed, spine straight, chest slightly sunk, knees slightly bent, and tailbone slightly tucked (imagine that you started sitting on a chair and then changed your mind; see fig. 5.5).

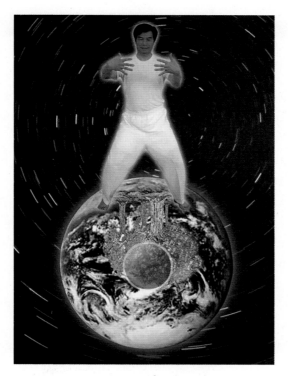

Figure 5.5. Beginning stance for this Chi Kung exercise.

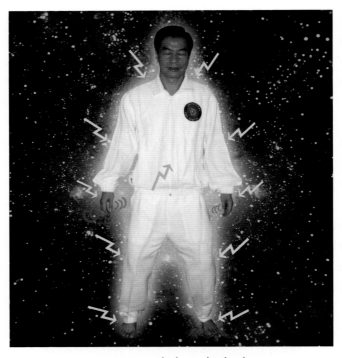

Figure 5.6. Shaking the body.

2. Take a deep breath, and as you let it out, relax. Repeat a few times. Now bring your attention to your abdominal area. Smile into your body.

3. Shake your body vigorously for one to two minutes from head to toes while keeping it pleasantly relaxed (fig. 5.6).

4. Stop and stand still, noticing the movement of chi in your body.

5. Focus on your navel and imagine there is a balloon right behind it. As you inhale, expand this balloon with a longer breath so that your abdomen expands.

6. As you exhale, shrink this balloon so that your navel is pulled inward toward the spine. The exhalation should be shorter than the inhalation.

7. Repeat the whole sequence of abdominal breathing either nine, eighteen, twenty-seven, or thirty-six times, then rest. Once you are comfortable with abdominal breathing, proceed to the next step.

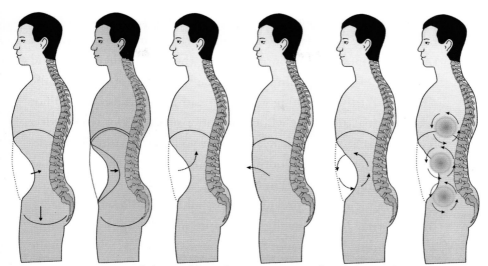

Figure 5.7. Abdominal breathing. Suction in the abdominal area draws chi into the skin.

8. This time you will do reverse abdominal breathing. This means that you will pull your navel toward your spine on the inhalation and relax your abdomen on the exhalation.

9. Repeat nine times. Pay attention to how you feel. When this way of breathing becomes comfortable, you can do eighteen, twenty-seven, or thirty-six repetitions.

10. You should practice reverse abdominal breathing until you can do it confidently, before proceeding to the next step.

11. Now you'll go back to normal abdominal breathing again. Inhale and expand your abdomen, then exhale all the air out, pulling your navel toward your spine as you exhale. Imagine that your navel is touching your spine. In this position, on the end of the exhale, you will hold your breath for a few seconds while visualizing the suction in your abdomen pulling chi in. Then, inhale and relax your abdomen. Repeat nine, eighteen, twenty-seven, or thirty-six times. Start with nine repetitions, then do more.

12. Rest and relax while you breathe very gently and naturally. As you breathe, bring your awareness to your skin. Feel your skin breathing.

13. When you gain enough confidence in this practice, you can add

the following modification. After completing reverse abdominal breathing from step 8 (either nine, eighteen, twenty-seven, or thirty-six times), hold your breath on the end of the exhale and begin to move your diaphragm as if you were attempting to breathe (Taoist call this "breathing without breathing" because you do not take in actual air). This will create more suction. Do it only for a few seconds at first, then relax and let your body naturally exhale. Then breathe naturally and imagine inhaling through your skin as well. Rest and feel your skin breathing.

14. After practicing the previous steps, add the following process: Imagine your lungs glowing with white metallic light and eventually expanding beyond your body's boundaries. Draw white metallic light into your skin pores while doing the skin breathing practice described above.

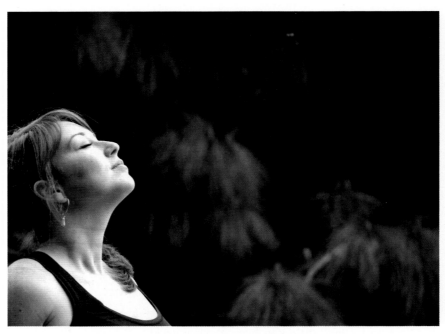

Figure 5.8. Skin Breathing in nature brings good clean Chi to skin and hair.

15. Finish the practice by smiling into your skin and taking a few deep, relaxing breaths. With practice you will develop a state of wonderful lightness and ease of breathing with your entire body.

This practice will leave you feeling energized, alive, and glowing with vitality. It will fill the skin with energy, clear carbon dioxide from the body, and bring more blood, oxygen, and nutrients into the skin.

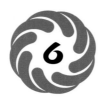

Vibrating the Body to Support Skin Stem Cells

Ancient Taoists believed that human beings are born immortal and then gradually lose this capability as a result of exposure to various harmful influences that waste their life force, accumulating damage as a result. It's easy to feel immortal and invincible when the body is young and healthy. And it's certainly true that the more damage and sickness the body accumulates, the more it loses its vibrancy, vitality, and beauty. For thousands of years, Taoist masters searched for the knowledge that would allow them to defy aging and stay vital and vibrant even in advanced age, and they developed a complete system of practices that cultivate longevity. Science now confirms that the Taoist idea of immortality is not so outlandish as it may seem.

Even though the physical body cannot stay young forever, even with the best possible care, it can be much more vibrant, agile, and radiant than most people believe, because there are cells in the human body, and in particular in the human skin, that can be maintained in a cell culture for hundreds of generations without losing their youth and vigor. These are the stem cells, and they are amazingly effective at regenerating the skin (as well as other areas of the body). To understand how stem cells

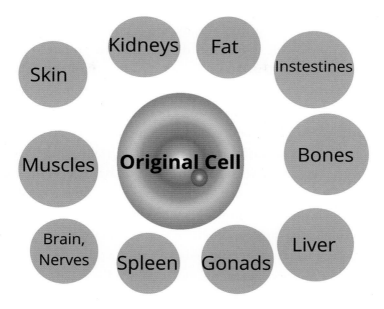

Figure 6.1. The very first cell of the human body is the mother of all cells.

work is to understand how to maintain and enhance the skin's beauty and vitality.

CELLS OF IMMORTALITY

Every human being begins as a single cell created by the union of a female egg and a male sperm. This first "mother of all cells" is *totipotent,* which means it can give birth to all the different cells in the human body and to the cells that make up the placenta and the umbilical cord.

This state of totipotency exists only for a short while before the cells start selecting their paths of development. From then on they are called *pluripotent cells.* Every cell in a fetus in utero is pluripotent. Fetal skin has the remarkable ability to regenerate without scarring or inflammation. Embryonic stem cells can be considered immortal, because when placed in a cell culture they can divide indefinitely without aging.

By the time the baby is born, most of the cells in its body are committed cells, which means they already have a predetermined fate. This means that they divide, grow, and differentiate to produce only one specific cell type, which can be a nerve cell, a blood cell, an epidermal cell, and so forth. They cannot change the course of their development. These cells have a limited life span. They eventually wear out, accumulate damage, and become less and less functional. Finally, they stop making any positive contribution to the overall health of the organ to which they belong and have to be destroyed. For example, in the epidermis, keratinocytes start as small, round cells residing on the basal membrane, and then they start growing, maturing, and moving toward the surface, accumulating protein keratin, which eventually replaces all their essential parts, including their nucleus, so that the cells cease to be alive and turn into protective keratinous scales. When these cells accumulate wear and tear, they slough off the skin's surface to make room for new keratinous scales, which eventually follow the same fate. Not all skin cells have such a brutal fate, but all of them follow this predetermined route—from a young and vital cell to an old and worn-out cell that self-destructs and is replaced by a new cell.

And yet in every tissue, including the skin, there is also a pool of direct descendants of the original immortal cells; these are the adult stem cells. These cells are *multipotent,* which means that under normal conditions they serve as a pool for replacing the cells that have been lost in the course of normal living. Stem cells are very slowly dividing cells. As they slowly divide, they replenish their own ranks while maintaining their regenerative powers. And if there is any kind of wound or injury, adult stem cells can transform themselves into multiple kinds of cells to ensure repair and regeneration.

One of the main reasons why cells age and die is because their replication is limited by telomeres, which are repetitive and nonsensical DNA sequences on the terminal end of a chromosome. As cells divide, telomeres become shorter and shorter. The shorter the telomere, the more aged and dysfunctional the cell. Embryonic and cancer cells escape this fate by using a special enzyme called *telomerase,* which keeps repairing the

Damage

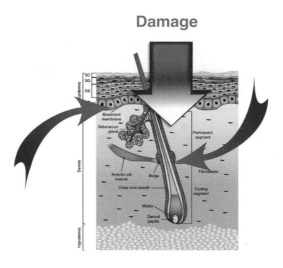

Figure 6.2. In case of an injury, the skin stem cells activate
and repair the skin.

shortened telomere, restoring its length. So only cancer cells and embryonic cells can be considered immortal and can be maintained in a cell culture indefinitely, provided they are given everything they need. Yet stem cells are very close to being immortal too because their telomeres do not shorten as fast as the telomeres in other cells. In an ideal world they should be able to repair and regenerate the body until a very old age, over a hundred years at least. In the real world, however, they lose energy, accumulate damage, and slowly lose their ability to repair tissues. Skin stem cells are especially vulnerable to damage and energy depletion because the skin is exposed to so many harmful environmental and chemical influences (and in many cases this includes cosmetic products).

There are three different types of adult stem cells found in the skin:

- **Epidermal stem cells:** These are located in the lowest layer of the epidermis. They are slowly dividing cells that are attached to a structure called the *basal membrane,* which separates the dermis from the epidermis and provides support and nutrition for epidermal stem cells.

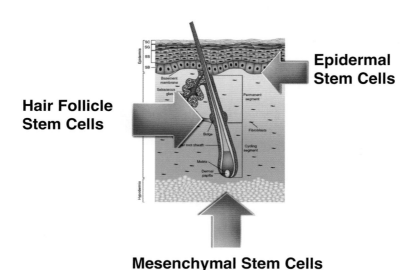

Epidermal Stem Cells

Hair Follicle Stem Cells

Mesenchymal Stem Cells

Figure 6.3. There are three different types of stem cells in the skin.

- **Hair follicle stem cells:** These are found inside the hair follicles, in a structure called the *bulge.* They can migrate out of the bulge to repair the skin.
- **Mesenchymal stem cells:** These are located in the underlying fat tissue. They are adult stem cells and can differentiate into various skin cells in case of an injury. They also can produce anti-inflammatory molecules and growth factors. Today researchers are actively investigating their use in skin repair and rejuvenation.

In 1991, Howard Green, professor emeritus at Harvard University and a pioneer in the science of skin regeneration, started using epidermal stem cells to help burn patients regenerate their own skin. He was able to save the lives of two children who had burns on over 90 percent of their body, which is commonly a fatal condition. Later, scientists learned how to engineer skin stem cells and subsequently used this technology to successfully replace the entire epidermis of a child who suffered from the genetic skin disease *Epidermolysis bullosa,* in which the skin and mucous membranes blister easily. All this demonstrates that the skin's stem cells are a gold reserve, and activating their powers of regeneration is the key to achieving younger-looking and more radiant skin.

The outcome of plastic surgery, cosmetic fillers, chemical peeling, laser resurfacing, and other such intense procedures greatly depends on the skin's ability to bounce back after an injury. This means good chi, good hydration, minimum toxins, reduced stress, proper nutrition with adequate absorption of nutrients, good circulation, and active stem cells. Even the best cosmetic products, trained professionals, and the most advanced procedure can fail if the skin has lost its ability to regenerate. Modern cosmetic remedies and procedures can do wonders, and they can stimulate repair and regeneration, balance skin chemistry, add more moisture, and protect the skin from harmful environmental influences. However, no cosmetic product will work if the skin's chi is depleted.

As well, most cosmetic products do not go deep enough to reach the skin's stem cells—which is a good thing because many ingredients in cosmetic products are damaging to living cells and can deplete the stem cells' chi. Taoist practices are safe for the skin because they beautify it from the inside out and from the outside in. Practicing Skin-Breathing Chi Kung (chapter 5) and Stem Cell Chi Kung (this chapter) can make a person feel more alive and alert and prevent age-related sluggishness and loss of vitality. These practices keep the skin detoxed and provide good circulation and active stem cells. They are the most powerful practices you can do for your skin, comparable to a daily application of the best antiaging cream on the market. The best part is that it's totally free.

THE OXYGEN PARADOX

In the previous chapter we looked at how important it is that the skin breathes. But as it turns out, oxygenating the skin may not always be a good idea. The reason Taoist holistic approaches are so valuable is because they have been developed with diligent attention to one's own body and its changes. As Western science has discovered, oxygen is a double-edged sword when it comes to skin regeneration. Yes, the skin needs oxygen because it needs energy. At the same time, too much oxygen can be toxic to stem cells. This is the "oxygen paradox." Oxygen is essential because cells use it to generate electromagnetic energy; oxygen is also toxic because in the process of generating energy, the cells produce highly reactive free radicals of oxygen, which can damage cellular membranes, proteins, and DNA, thereby accelerating aging.

Stem cells are hidden away in specialized "rooms" called *stem cell niches.* These are anatomical structures that protect the stem cells and separate them from the surrounding tissues. Most stem cell niches have slightly lower oxygen content compared to the rest of the body's tissues. In inhaled air, ambient oxygen tension is 21 percent. By the time it reaches the tissues, it drops considerably. Partial oxygen pressure in most tissues is measured to be between 2 and 9 percent. However, in stem cell niches, partial oxygen pressure can be even lower, from 1 to 6 percent. Since stem cells do not do much, they are on an oxygen "diet" to protect them from free-radical damage.

This system works really well when the skin is young; however skin aging brings with it a number of unfavorable conditions. First, the skin's circulation becomes less efficient, depriving stem cells of oxygen even more than usual. Second, toxins and damage accumulate with age, disrupting the stem cells' ability to activate. Third, the water content in the skin diminishes due to the reduced water-holding capacity of aging skin. Less water means less favorable conditions for skin cell communication, movement, and toxic waste removal. As a result, the skin's stem cells become progressively dormant and inactive. Increasing their oxygen supply will activate them, but giving them too much, too fast may actually damage them.

WRINKLES AND THE STEM CELL PARADOX

The skin has a complex architecture. Its upper layer, the epidermis, has a layered structure and consists of cells at different stages of maturity. From baby cells residing in the depths of the epidermis, to the horny top layer, or stratum corneum, where flat, fully mature, hardened keratinous scales shield the body from elements with their protein-filled bodies, the epidermis is a marvel of nature's ingenuity. The dermis is very different from the epidermis and it too has an orderly and structured architecture comprised of sturdy networks of collagen and elastin embedded in a gel-like substance that ensures the smoothness, suppleness, and resilience of the skin.

When the skin begins to age, it still has the same complex architecture, but this architecture now has many faulty areas that create lines and wrinkles and uneven relief on the skin's surface. For example, the aging epidermis has areas where old, damaged cells refuse to move on, and so they accumulate, creating mottled pigmentation and roughness. The dermis has areas where old collagen is fused together and tangled into amorphous masses that no longer provide resilience and support. One of the most noticeable changes in the subcutaneous layer is the gradual loss of fat. This thinning of the fat layer makes the skin appear less plump and can lead to a more "hollowed" or "sunken" appearance, particularly under the eyes or in the cheeks. This loss of fat can also make wrinkles more noticeable. This is why people who have a thicker layer of subcutaneous fat may have fewer wrinkles compared to those who started with a thinner layer of fat. In addition, blood vessels may become more fragile and prone to damage, leading to the formation of small bruises (purpura) or red spots on the skin. Loss of elasticity in the subcutaneous fascia, due to damaged collagen and elastin, can lead to skin sagging. Fat may accumulate under the chin or form a pouch in the lower part of the abdomen due to sagging skin and the forces of gravity. For the skin to remain healthy, vibrant, and beautiful, all three layers have to be regularly renewed.

First, it is important to maintain renewal of the epidermis because it is the outermost layer of skin that is visible and also serves as the first line of defense. Second, the dermis has to be renewed because it provides resilience, smoothness, and support for the epidermis. And finally, the layer of subcutaneous fat and fascia has to be healthy and replenished because it protects the inner organs and defines the contours of the face and body. Of course, since the skin is not separate from the rest of the body, all the organs need to be replenished and renewed and kept healthy and radiant in order for the skin to remain healthy and beautiful.

Many people associate aging with wrinkles. However not all wrinkles result from natural aging. Some of them start as symptoms of skin damage or lack of moisture. There are four types of wrinkles:

1. **Fine lines:** These are thin wrinkles that become more apparent when a person is tired or stressed. These wrinkles are the easiest to remove, at least temporarily. When the skin is well-hydrated, it looks younger and has a soft glow that masks such fine wrinkles.

2. **Expression wrinkles:** These wrinkles first appear on the forehead, around the eyes (where they are called crow's feet), and at the sides of the mouth (where they are called smile lines or frown lines). They are created by the muscles pulling and stretching the skin. To eliminate these kinds of wrinkles, many women get injections of the botulinum toxin, one of the most poisonous biological substances known, which blocks electricity flowing through the skin's nerves, effectively paralyzing the site of the injection. These injections have to be repeated; for example, in the case of Botox, it may be required every four months since the nerves restore their conductivity in that amount of time. The main problem with this approach is that it does not restore the skin's elasticity and resilience, nor does it regenerate or rejuvenate the skin. It works only on expression wrinkles and only temporarily. Then there is the loss of one's natural facial expressions due to paralyzed facial muscles, which creates challenges when it comes to communicating with others.

3. **Sagging and loose skin:** These wrinkles develop as a result of the gradual stretching of the skin and weakening of its structures. Surgeons solve this problem by cutting off the excess skin and tightening up the remaining part. This is what's involved in a surgical face-lift, and it is a very efficient method of removing flaps and folds. With a face-lift you can achieve tight skin that looks

great from a distance. However a face-lift does not change the structure of the skin, it merely tightens it.

4. **Wrinkles from underlying damage:** The skin accumulates damage with age. The main factor is UV radiation. When the skin's collagen and elastin are damaged, its surface becomes uneven, with dimpled, bumpy areas. UV-induced skin damage is called *photoaging* and can produce deep, coarse wrinkles, mottled pigmentation, and elastosis, which is the result of prolonged and excessive sun exposure.

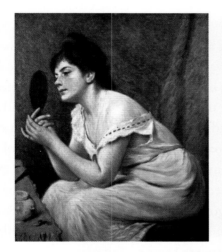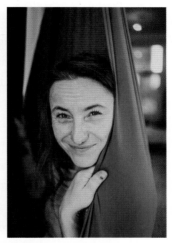

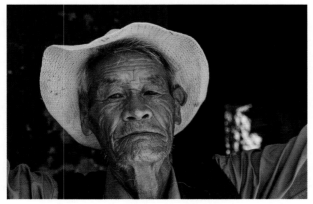

Figure 6.4. Types of wrinkles: a) fine lines, as in the painting *The First Wrinkle*, by Federico Zandomeneghi; b) expression wrinkles; c) wrinkles from sun damage and sagging skin.

When it comes to renovating and remodeling a building, it is often necessary to demolish faulty and damaged structures because they are impossible to repair. In the same way, many structures in aging skin accumulate so much damage and become so dysfunctional that they have to be destroyed and replaced with new structures. Since ancient times people have noticed that after an injury the skin often starts looking remarkably younger. In olden times, women who wanted to stop skin aging would sometimes use hot ash from the fireplace, vinegar, or other acids to burn away old skin in the hopes of regaining youth and radiance. Sadly this often resulted in scarring and skin infections.

Today we know that adding a bit of external damage can serve as a wake-up call for the skin, activating the mechanisms responsible for demolishing old structures and building new ones. There is no need to burn one's face with vinegar, though, because the cosmetics industry has developed many safe and effective methods for inflicting the kind of very mild damage that can activate stem cells and stimulate skin regeneration. However many people who use such products and procedures for rejuvenation often do not realize that they may be at risk of exhausting their skin's gold reserve. No cosmetic product or procedure can rejuvenate and renew the skin. They can only stimulate regeneration.

Here is where it's important to consider the stem cell paradox. To stay young and capable of regenerating skin, stem cells have to be kept in a sleepy and relaxed state as much as possible to preserve their life force. The more they are forced to work in emergency situations, which is what happens in a case of encouraging damage to the skin, the more they are at risk of exhausting their chi. Any damage that goes too deep will create inflammation and stress, and any damage that is too mild and superficial will not produce noticeable results. So the ideal approach would be to stimulate the skin in a holistic way, which helps the stem cells regain their regenerative powers yet does not create too much stress and inflammation.

CONTROLLED DAMAGE IN COSMETOLOGY

Today those who want to look younger and more beautiful have many choices—so many that it's easy to be overwhelmed with the profusion of promises of quick rejuvenation. However quick is not always better. Because the skin is a complex biological structure, with many different types of cells all connected to the entire body, anything that produces a fast and impressive result is probably coming with a price, and this price is not only financial.

Types of Controlled Damage Used to Stimulate Skin Renewal

- **Scrubs:** These are cosmetic products that contain abrasive particles that remove dead cells from skin's surface. Some scrubs contain soft polyethylene granules and others may have rough, hard particles such as finely ground almond shells, coffee, salt, or sugar. Scrubs remove only the very upper layer of cornified cells and do not damage the living layers of the epidermis; however people with thin and sensitive skin may experience skin irritation.

- **Chemical exfoliators such as alpha- and beta-hydroxy acids:** These kinds of products remove dead skin cells by dissolving the "glue" that holds them together. Acids also activate enzymes that accelerate natural skin renewal, so the skin starts looking younger. Alpha-hydroxy acid (AHA) products have different concentrations of acid. For example, alpha-hydroxy acid products sold over the counter exfoliate only the very upper layer of the stratum corneum and rarely cause any discomfort, except perhaps in those with extremely sensitive skin. With regular use, alpha-hydroxy acids help stimulate renewal in the epidermis and have little or no effect on the dermis. Beta hydroxy acids (BHAs) are a class of organic compounds commonly used in skincare products due to their exfoliating and pore-cleansing properties. The most well-known BHA is salicylic acid, which is derived from willow bark.

BHAs are similar to AHAs in their exfoliating effects but have some distinct differences. They possess anti-inflammatory properties and they are soluble in oils, which makes them well-suited for unclogging pores and treating oily and acne-prone skin.

- **Dermabrasion and microdermabrasion:** These methods mechanically remove the upper layer of the epidermis. Dermabrasion causes deeper damage and requires a longer recovery time. Microdermabrasion "polishes" the skin by creating a fast-moving stream of abrasive particles. It is a less invasive method, with easier recovery. This type of damage affects the skin on a deeper level compared to scrubs and alpha-hydroxy acids; however renewing the dermis remains a challenge.

- **Lasers:** These are light-emitting devices that completely destroy the upper layer of skin. One version is ablative carbon dioxide lasers, which heat up water in the epidermis so fast it evaporates,

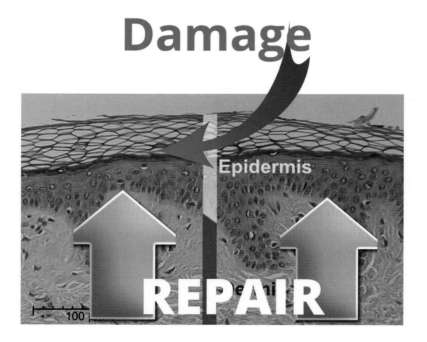

Figure 6.5. Controlled damage activates skin renewal.

destroying (ablating) living cells. In the underlying layer of the dermis, collagen is coagulated, which produces a tightening effect and stimulates the formation of new collagen. This produces the most astonishing rejuvenation but requires a long period of healing. Other types of lasers ablate the skin selectively, leaving the surrounding areas intact, which shortens the recovery period but the effect is less impressive.

In addition to these methods, the cosmetics industry continuously develops new approaches. Still, scrubs and chemical exfoliators remain the most popular method of skin exfoliation because they are safe and easy to use at home. Scrubs containing salt and hard abrasives such as almond shell are usually used for body exfoliation, while scrubs containing soft polyethylene granules are used for facial skin. In a typical at-home product containing alpha-hydroxy acids, the maximum concentration of such acids never exceeds 10 percent, and for beta-hydroxy acids (salicylic acid) it is no more than 2 percent. The most popular are glycolic, lactic, citric, malic, tartaric, and phytic acids. Glycolic acid has the smallest molecule size, is the most popular, and can penetrate deep into the skin. Next comes lactic acid, which is naturally found in sour milk and also naturally present in human skin. Professional beauty salons can use stronger exfoliators such as higher concentrations of glycolic acids and other alpha-hydroxy acids with 30 to 70 percent of alpha-hydroxy acids and 20 to 30 percent of salicylic acid. They are still considered surface peelings, but they burn deeper into the epidermis.

Next are medium peels such as trichloroacetic acid (TCA) peels. This is an analog of the acetic acid found in vinegar, in which the three hydrogen atoms of the methyl group have all been replaced by chlorine atoms. And then there are the deep peels, or phenol peels, which produce the best rejuvenation effects compared to other chemical exfoliators, but also are associated with a longer recovery time and greater risk. These methods can be used as an emergency method to remove accumulated damage, but they should be used with caution.

Whether we are talking about chemical peels, lasers, dermabrasion, or other methods of controlled damage, the deeper the damage, the more impressive the rejuvenation, yet also the more discomfort, higher cost, greater risk, and longer recovery. Still, many people believe that achieving a much younger and more vibrant-looking skin is worth it. What many do not realize is that all methods of controlled damage, even the most advanced and newest forms, can only help the skin get rid of the damage; they do not repair and rejuvenate the skin. The actual task of restoration and regeneration is done by silent and invisible workers within the skin, the stem cells. They are the cells that replenish and rebuild the skin, restoring its original architecture and producing the desired rejuvenating effects.

When the stem cells are active and vital, controlled skin damage yields a glowing and healthy skin. If, however, the stem cells are weak and inactive, applying any of these methods will not produce the same result and may lead to a long and arduous recovery, inflammation, scarring, and discoloration. And as pointed out, many methods that provide fast and impressive skin rejuvenation through controlled skin damage also risk exhausting the stem cells' chi. So when it comes to maintaining your skin's health, vitality, and radiance throughout your lifetime, taking care of your stem cells and making sure any interventions are safe and as close to natural regeneration as possible must be a top priority.

THE NEED FOR DEEPER HYDRATION

Essential to skin renewal is proper hydration. Well-hydrated skin not only immediately looks plumper, suppler, and more attractive, it also regenerates much better. We all know that covering a wound with a dressing keeps the wound moist, accelerates healing, and greatly reduces the risk of scarring. However skin is not all that easy to hydrate. For example, just drinking more water or splashing water on the skin will not make much of a difference in its hydration. Human skin, just like skin of all terrestrial organisms, evolved to prevent living bodies from drying out in the sun and swelling with too much water in the rain or during a swim. This means that the skin is naturally very good at preventing water from crossing the boundary that protects the interior of the body.

Skin prevents water from entering the body and yet skin itself needs water to function. Since the epidermis does not have its own blood vessels, water from the inside of the body (which is replenished by drinking water) has to migrate into the dermis. Driven by the differences (or gradient) in water content (it is drier on the surface), water moves through the dermis toward the epidermis, and then it evaporates. Picture a continuous flow of water that keeps the skin hydrated: it moves from the watery environment inside the body to the moist dermis to the much drier epidermis and then to the even drier air on the outside. When cosmetic products block the evaporation of water from the surface, they do help skin preserve water and the skin temporarily does become more hydrated and therefore it does look noticeably younger. However, the danger of this is that if such products are used too often, the overhydrated upper layer will not provide the important moisture gradient and this will reduce the natural movement of moisture and therefore may lead to drier skin and more noticeable wrinkles.

The skin does have structures that allow it to conserve water. The main barrier that prevents evaporation is the stratum corneum, the horny or cornified layer that consists of dead, hard, flat, keratinous scales. These protein-rich cells provide some protection from dryness, but not enough to allow the skin to stay smooth, soft, and radiant. Keratinous scales do not just prevent moisture from leaving the skin, they also attract water to the skin's surface. This is possible because each cell in the stratum corneum is covered with molecules that have what's known as a *natural moisturizing factor,* or NMF. These molecules attract water from moisture in the environment and bind it to the skin's surface, keeping keratinous scales soft, moist, and flexible. If the NMF is washed away as happens when we wash the skin with hot (not warm) water or use drying soaps or chemicals, the skin may become drier. So one way to help the skin retain water is by replacing lost NMF. Many moisturizers on the market mimic NMF, but those who want to restore

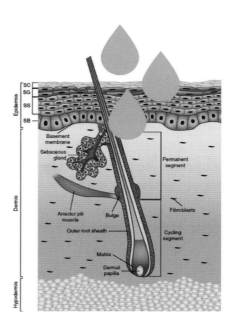

Figure 6.6. The stratum corneum can attract water from the air.

the skin's vibrancy and beauty need to start looking much deeper and understand what it really takes to restore the skin's radiance through deep hydration.

In the past it was believed that the stratum corneum had a "bricks-and-mortar" structure in which hard, keratinous scales are glued together by skin oil. In this model, the cornified cells provide a mechanical barrier (the "bricks"), while skin oil (the "mortar") makes sure they stay together to prevent water from evaporating from the epidermis. Since then, more detailed studies have revealed that the oily "mortar" between keratinous scales is different from the sebum found on the skin's surface because it does not come from the sebaceous glands and consists of different kinds of lipids, called *ceramides*. Each ceramide molecule has a water-soluble "head" made of a chemical compound called *sphingosine* and a lipid-soluble "tail" made of long-chained polyunsaturated fatty acids. When immersed in water, all "heads" group together to stay immersed and all "tails" group together, creating multilayered sheets of lipid bilayers and water between keratinous scales in the stratum corneum. The resulting structure is reminiscent of a Russian Napoleon cake, which is made with layers of puff pastry with creamy filling between the layers, only in the skin it is layers of waterproofing lipids with microscopically thin layers of water in between. It is interesting that when scientists investigated the resulting structures closer, they discovered that they form multiple layers of crystalline structures. First, ceramides are organized into a very orderly, crystal-like structure, and next, water, sandwiched between lipid bilayers, turned out to be organized in crystal-like structures as well. Finally, even the protein keratin inside every cornified cell has a crystal-like structure. The skin's surface, therefore, is full of biological crystals!

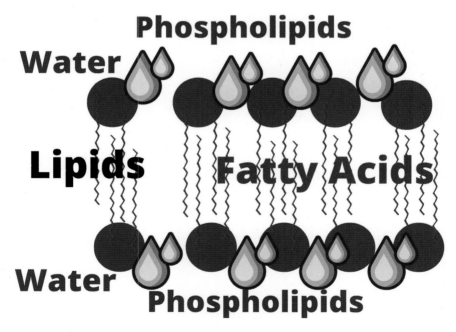

Figure 6.7. The epidermis has lipid structures that preserve water and work as biological crystals to amplify chi and create radiance.

Even young skin will look dull and less vital if it does not shine from within. To shine, the skin has to have a healthy, well-structured, crystaline "mask" that radiates one's essence out into the world. The human body is not only wrapped in skin, it is also protected by the skin's biological crystals, which can modify electromagnetic energy such as light. This is what liquid crystals do in the skin, in addition to preserving moisture. When a person's face lights up, looking radiant and glowing, it's not just a trick of the imagination—it's the effects of the skin's crystals amplifying and radiating one's personal energy, or chi. Hot water, detergents, soaps, and alcohol-based cleansers can damage the crystaline structure of the skin. When this happens, the skin becomes dull, lifeless, and often develops irritations and blemishes, and with the loss of its radiant layer the skin also loses its glow. According to the Tao, a person's radiance starts in the heart and then radiates out through the skin.

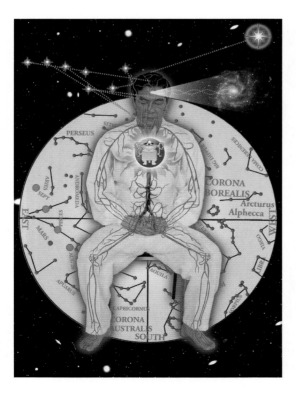

Figure 6.8. The heart radiance amplifies into the skin and expresses itself outwardly.

Epidermal lipids are not produced by the skin's sebaceous glands. Instead they are released from the maturing epidermal cells right before they give up their life to become the dead, cornified cells of the stratum corneum. This means that renewal of the epidermal lipid crystals goes hand in hand with the renewal of the entire epidermis. All living cells need water. Since the epidermis does not have its own blood vessels, the hydration of the epidermis goes along with the renewal and stimulation of blood and lymphatic circulation of the dermis. Therefore deep hydration helps skin renewal and provides radiance.

VIBRATIONS FOR STEM CELL REJUVENATION

Today scientists believe that it is possible to keep the stem cells younger and more active by taking care of their microenvironment, or "niche." This calls for a gentle and holistic approach. The Tao regards every organ's health to be the result of the harmonious teamwork of all the organs in the body. First and foremost, it is important to keep the skin and the body in general as toxin-free as possible, because toxins can inhibit or damage stem cells. Second, it is important to supply the stem cells with oxygen, nutrients, and growth factors. Third, stem cells have to receive enough energy to stay active in order to be able to repair tissues. This means that to keep the skin vital and radiant, it is not enough to simply destroy old tissue and wait for stem cells to come to the rescue. We also need to stimulate both the blood circulation and the lymphatic flow, which removes toxins and delivers the building blocks necessary for skin regeneration, oxygenization, and the growth factors necessary for skin renewal.

Another benefit achieved by the stimulation of the blood and lymphatic flow is the resulting hydration. The epidermis does not have its own blood vessels and receives its hydration from the blood vessels in the dermis, which makes it dependent on dermal circulation. This is where Taoist practices excel, as one's focused awareness helps bring more electromagnetic energy to the area of the body on which one's attention is focused, and relaxation is important for switching the body into the parasympathetic mode, which supports regeneration and counteracts the exhaustion of stem cells as a result of stress.

From a holistic, body-mind-soul-spirit perspective, every organ needs love and chi in order to remain vital. All these goals can be achieved with Stem Cell Chi Kung practice, which is easy to learn and completely safe. This form of Chi Kung has been practiced by Taoist masters for thousands of years, long before anybody knew anything about stem cells. It includes relaxation, awareness, mindfulness, and intentional breathing, combined with vibrational stimulation of the skin. As described in the following exercise, applying gentle vibrations delivered by a bamboo hitter or your own palms can bring deeper and more lasting hydration to the skin compared to the moisturization achieved by skin-care products alone.

Stem Cell Chi Kung with Bamboo Hitter

Using a bamboo hitter or your own palms to deliver gentle vibrations allows you to achieve renewal and hydration on a deep level, without the use of chemical compounds. This is one of the easiest and simplest approaches to radiance and beauty. For this practice you will need a bamboo hitter or an equivalent that is capable of delivering gentle vibrations; alternately, you can use your own palms. It is very important that the slapping action is gentle enough so as not to cause any bruising or pain, but energetic enough to create vibrations. This practice can be combined with Inner Smile Chi Kung, described in chapter 4 (p. 71), and Skin-Breathing Chi Kung, described in chapter 5 (p. 82).

Note: Do not use a bamboo hitter right after using peeling agents, scrubs, or any other skin treatment that temporarily makes the skin more vulnerable. However, this kind of stimulation is a great way to prepare your skin for more intensive cosmetic procedures.

1. Stand in Chi Kung posture, your feet shoulder-width apart, shoulders relaxed, knees slightly bent and positioned approximately over your toes, tailbone slightly tucked, spine upright.

2. Relax, take a deep breath, and as you exhale, smile.

3. Slowly and gently shake your entire body. Move your attention from your feet to your ankles, to your thighs, your abdomen, up your spine, and through your arms and fingers.

4. If you're going to use your hands to lightly hit your body, rub your palms together to make them warm and energized. Breathe and smile.

5. Standing, feel your feet connected to the earth and your crown connected to the universe. Take a deep breath and relax. Smile into your heart and feel your heart smiling at you.

6. Become aware of your spine. Locate the point directly across from your navel on your spine, as shown in figure 6.9. This is called the Door of Life. It is a very important energy center that in the Taoist tradition is believed to be connected to the regeneration of the body.

7. Using either a bamboo hitter or your own hands, lightly tap your Door of Life. Even a few minutes of this practice is enough to activate skin. Listen to your body to determine when you have awakened your skin sufficiently. It should feel warm, alive, and open.

8. Stop and breathe into your Door of Life. Smile and relax.

9. Next, you can add the abdominal breathing and skin breathing practices. Begin abdominal breathing, repeating nine times: expand your abdomen on the inhalation, and then shrink it on the exhalation, pulling your navel toward your spine. (For a review, see chapter 5, p. 84.)

10. Do reverse abdominal breathing nine times, pulling your navel toward your spine on the inhalation and expanding your abdomen on the exhalation. At this point you can include a few minutes of skin breathing. Rest before moving to the next step.

11. Inhale, then this time, on the exhale, hold your breath and mentally push your chi into your Door of Life, feeling it expanding. While still holding your breath and keeping the back of your body expanded, gently hit your Door of Life a few times and then exhale and relax. Expanding your back with chi and holding your breath on the top of the inhale while gently hitting helps create kidney vibrations which help awaken the kidneys.

12. Stretch out your right arm and gently hit your skin from the fingers to your shoulder with a bamboo hitter or using your other palm. The hits should be gentle so as not to cause any pain or discomfort. Aim for skin vibration. Then continue hitting your skin across your body toward the left leg and work on your leg from the thigh to the toes (sitting down if necessary).

13. Repeat the same process with the left arm and right leg. Then hit the back of your thighs and your buttocks.

14. Gently hit your chest and your back. Gently work on your scalp and face with gentle tapping movements of your fingertips or the tips of the bamboo hitter.

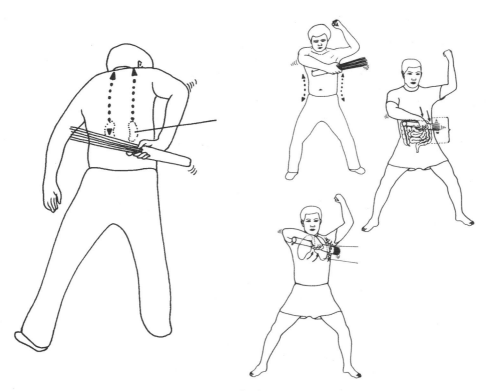

Figure 6.9. LEFT: Stem Cell Chi Kung with a bamboo
hitter on the Door of Life.
RIGHT: Using a bamboo hitter on body points on
the arms, torso, and legs.

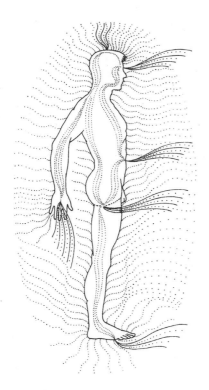

Figure 6. 10. The skin is stimulated by vibration, which increases circulation and hydration.

15. Finish with chi massage: rub your hands together and move them without touching your skin over your face, head, neck, chest, abdomen, and legs.
16. Take a deep breath and smile. Finish with the Inner Smile, described in chapter 4, which can be done standing up, seated, or even lying down.

This practice makes your skin feel energized, awakened, and alive. Gentle vibration reaches deep into the dermis and underlying fat and muscle tissues, stimulating lymphatic and blood circulation, loosening fibrous walls between fat cells, bringing deeper awareness to the body, and directing more electromagnetic energy to the skin. As a result, the stem cell environment becomes cleaner, more oxygenated, more hydrated, and more nutrient-rich. Remember that this hitting practice must be done gently and with full awareness. Inner focus is important. Keep your body relaxed and remember to smile throughout the practice. Drink plenty of purified water to help flush out the toxins removed by lymphatic flow.

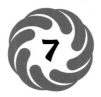

Beauty and Emotions

Imagination is the beginning of creation. You imagine what you desire, you will what you imagine, and at last you create what you will.

GEORGE BERNARD SHAW

The skin is closely connected to the nervous system. In embryogenesis, i.e., the formation of the embryo, the nervous system and the skin (the epidermis, sebaceous glands, and hair follicles) all originate from the same source, the ectoderm, the outermost of the three primary layers of an embryo that is the source of various tissues and structures (*ecto* means "external"). Together with the nervous system, the skin responds to the energies of the outer universe and expresses the energies of the inner universe to the outside world. Thus it is only natural that the skin is influenced by the nervous system and is affected by thoughts, emotions, and the energy of the mind. This influence can be detrimental or beneficial, incidental or intentional, momentary or long-lasting.

THE PERSONALITY MASK

The skin registers sensations that can be internal or external; it expresses emotions and is affected by emotional energies physically, chemically, and physiologically. Facial skin is especially affected by the emotions

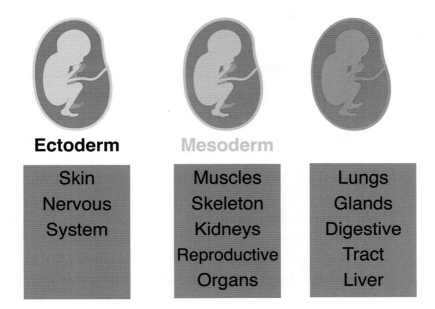

Figure 7.1. The skin and the nervous system originate from the same source, the ectoderm, during embryogenesis.

because our face expresses our feelings. Smiling, frowning, laughing, and crying are just a few examples of outward expressions of the emotions, which inevitably pull, stretch, and move the skin of the face. When people are young, their skin is very resilient and will easily return to its original condition. With age, however, the skin's structural proteins, collagen and elastin, start weakening, so it takes a little while longer for aged skin to relax the wrinkles that occur from frowning or smiling. Eventually, though, wrinkles stay and accumulate. Habitual feelings, once stored in the skin, create a characteristic personality mask. People do not have a choice as to whether or not they will develop a personality mask, but they can take actions to ensure that their personality mask expresses their most beautiful aspects.

Factors That Affect the Personality Mask

- **Amount of underlying damage:** The stronger and more resilient the skin's collagen and elastin, the easier it is for the skin to relax wrinkles and other emotional expressions. The more damage collagen and elastin accumulate, the less capable they are of returning the skin back to its original appearance. Because the skin is an organ that is continuously affected by gravity, downward expressions such as grief, displeasure, sadness, upset, and disappointment will alter the skin more because these expressions are reinforced by the downward action of gravity. Smiling and other upward expressions naturally create a more uplifted expression, but they need to be practiced more to produce this effect since they have to work against gravity.

- **Skin regeneration:** Insufficient regeneration leads to deeper wrinkles and more of a downward expression due to the force of gravity slowly pulling the skin down. This means that even if your mood is always neutral, natural forces of gravity and aging will tend to create a downward expression. To counteract this, the Tao suggests practicing smiling and joyful uplifting expressions intentionally.

- **Skin hydration:** The skin's resilience is created not only by collagen and elastin, but also by the water-holding gel of glycosaminoglycan in the dermis (see chapter 1). This creates a kind of waterbed that helps the skin stay smooth. The skin's fascia, which allows the facial muscles to move and stretch, needs lubrication in order to move with ease. Deep hydration achieved through improved blood and lymph circulation helps reduce expression wrinkles.

- **Holding on to the emotions:** People who have difficulty letting go are more likely to have one particular emotion (usually negative) ingrained in their skin as they age. Worry, anxiety, anger, resentment, and grief are examples of long-lasting emotions that may become an unwanted personality mask. Taoists advise releasing such emotions daily, regardless of where they came from, the same way people clean their houses or take showers daily.

- **Individual characteristics of the skin:** Thin skin will be more affected by the emotions, while thicker skin with a more robust dermal layer may be more resilient to stretching and pulling.

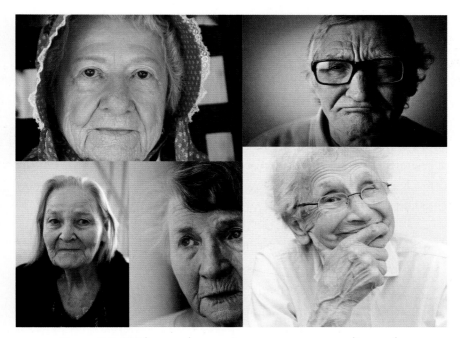

Figure 7.2. With age, the emotions create a personality mask.

THE COST OF HOLDING BACK EMOTIONS

Taoists understand that it is impossible to eliminate *all* negative emotions. In fact, it would be very unwise. Biologically and evolutionarily, painful and unpleasant feelings are chemical communications from our body to the brain that tell the brain to pay close attention. For example, fear is an important emotion that keeps us alive by stopping us from doing something dangerous, while physical pain is an important sensation that makes sure we do not ignore an open wound or a broken bone. Because negative emotions have been so important for our survival, they tend to outweigh positive emotions, and they also grow much faster. Taoists advise maintaining balance by clearing negative emotions daily. It is important to mention that the energy-clearing practices presented in this book are designed only for helping skin stay more radiant and beautiful. They are not designed for dealing with childhood traumas or any emotion that has to be processed before releasing.

In the Taoist tradition, negative emotions are comparable to weeds in the garden that do not need help to grow, while positive and virtuous emotions are like flowers that require love and care to grow.

Taoist masters discovered that balancing the emotional energies in the body is the key to youth, radiance, and longevity. Since negative emotions are very easy to come by, they have to be regularly released from the body, as holding on to negative emotions indefinitely will accelerate aging and make the body more vulnerable to illness. On the other hand, positive emotions are often short-lived and need to be nurtured and replenished.

The Physical Results of Holding on to Negative Emotions

- **Chronic muscle tension:** In addition to creating an unpleasant personality mask, unprocessed negative emotions can create chronic muscle tension that blocks energy flow and impedes skin circulation. On a systemic level this tension interferes with breathing and energy flow throughout the body.

- **Inflammation:** Negative emotions that are not released from the body have been linked to chronic, low-grade inflammation in tissues. As previously noted, the term *inflammaging* describes the process of aging caused by chronic inflammation. Chronic unhappiness and stress creates inflammation not only in the skin, but in all the organs and organ systems.

- **Impeded regeneration:** Chronic stress and anxiety depletes the body's energy reserves, restricts breathing, and constricts skin capillaries, impairing circulation.

- **Diminished radiance:** When people are wrapped up in negative thoughts and emotions, it blocks the skin's luminosity. Words such as *gloomy, dreary, shadowy,* and *drab* describe the grim state of skin when there are persistent negative emotions. This may be the result of the combined effects of insufficient hydration caused by blocked circulation, low oxygen, and blocked energy flow.

MOLECULES OF JOY

Taoist masters long ago discovered what we all know intuitively: positive and happy feelings have rejuvenating and invigorating effects on the body, while negative, toxic emotions, when their chemistry and energy accumulates in the body, can make a person sick and accelerate aging. Every emotion in the body has a unique chemical signature that determines its physiological effects. Emotions can be compared to prescriptions the mind gives to one's inner pharmacist. Some of them, such as joy, love, and gratitude, are like invigorating elixirs and vitamins. Others, such as sadness, anger, and fear, are like bitter medicine that may be necessary for survival, but should not be taken indefinitely because of their side effects. The skin is affected by more than a hundred neurochemicals that are released in response to all the various emotions. The "happy" ones are oxytocin, serotonin, dopamine, and the endorphins. Researchers have found that they are responsible for producing a youthful, luminous, vibrant, vital state of being, and this is reflected in the skin.[1]

Of the three endorphins found in humans, beta-endorphin, a peptide produced in the central and peripheral nervous systems (including the neurons of the skin) has a broad spectrum of physiological activity that affects mood, immune function, and pain level. The nervous system releases beta-endorphin when people are in love or feel pleasure, and also, paradoxically, in response to an injury, pain, and UV radiation. The reason beta-endorphin is released in response to pain is because it reduces pain. This is why those who have just suffered a serious accident often report euphoria in the immediate aftermath and not being aware of any pain until much later. Skin cells have receptors for beta-endorphin and therefore are affected by this regulatory peptide.

Beta-endorphin has a unique ability to stimulate an increase in the amount of nitric oxide in the body. This is a chemical compound that relaxes muscles in the blood vessels, opening them to flow, and this creates an instant beautifying and illuminating effect. The reason beta-endorphin can instantly illuminate the skin is because its radiance

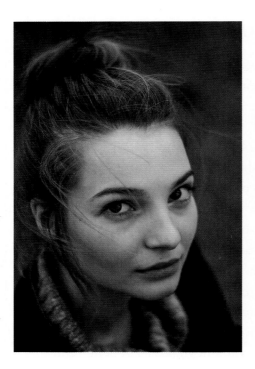

Figure 7.3. The capillary network in young skin is what creates a rosy glow.

greatly depends on the condition of the capillaries. In young skin, arterial capillaries in the upper dermis form a dense layer of capillary loops. In one square millimeter of skin on the face, there could be up to 150 such loops.

When light penetrates the epidermis and reflects this dense pillow of coiled blood vessels, it reflects back to the observer and creates that magical glow of youth. With age, and especially if a person is chronically stressed, the tiny capillaries in the face become smaller and thinner until they disappear altogether. The skin can still receive blood because of the presence of the larger blood vessels, which become even larger to compensate for the loss of small capillaries. As the damage from UV radiation and inflammation caused by stress and toxins creates low-grade chronic inflammation, the blood vessels in the skin may start forming spiderlike structures that lead to uneven redness of the skin. So instead of that smooth, uniform, rosy glow of youth, as we age we tend to develop red spots on the cheeks and chin, redness of the nose, and visibly enlarged veins under the skin.

Beta-endorphin and other biologically active molecules that are produced when we are happy and joyful (often described as "feel-good molecules") are the biological key that opens the way for the skin's regeneration. When the body is under stress and is in fight-or-flight mode, it directs blood and energy to the arms and legs as an evolutionary strategy for either fighting or running away, and to do so it constricts the skin's capillaries. This prevents excessive bleeding in case of an injury, but it also shuts down the skin's regeneration capabilities. Once the danger has passed, the body releases happy molecules so they can reopen the skin's capillaries and restore blood flow to the skin.

This is why those who are chronically stressed have a noticeable lack of radiance to their skin. Practices that help us switch off the fight-or-flight alarm and allow us to release happy chemistry cause the deep capillary loops in the dermis to relax, which allows the skin to rejuvenate. If you can keep your skin relaxed and saturated with molecules of joy, they will preserve and enhance your radiance. Today many companies are marketing skin-care products that promise stimulation of feel-good chemicals in the skin. Such products may contain cacao oil, Dead Sea salts, Panax ginseng, or other herbal extracts. However the best and surest way to increase feel-good chemistry in the skin is by cultivating positive emotions. In the Taoist tradition, intentional laughing and smiling into one's own organs are the foundational practices for health, beauty, and rejuvenation.

Other chemicals that have a positive effect on the skin are dopamine, which is produced when people feel good about their achievements; oxytocin, which is a love and bonding hormone; and serotonin, which is a pleasure, happiness, and relaxation hormone. They are all molecules of joy because when people feel loved, accomplished, happy, and relaxed all at once, they often describe this state as joy. Children naturally experience joy as their default state of being. A child may feel angry, frustrated, sad, afraid, or upset in the moment, but once the situation improves, they quickly return to joy and radiance. In contrast, most adults find joy a very rare guest.

Taoist masters of old discovered something that the modern personal development movement realized only in the second half of the twentieth century: the human mind can intentionally create love, joy, and happiness instead of waiting for external circumstances to get better. The formula for issuing such a happiness "prescription" for the skin includes physical relaxation, mindfulness, and creative visualization. Taoist masters teach that emotional energy is quite real. As we discussed in the previous chapters, science confirms that thoughts are clouds of electromagnetic energy resulting from electricity moving through the physical "wires" that are the body's nerves. When the electromagnetic current moves through the nerves, neurons release neurochemicals, which produce physiological effects. What people perceive as an emotion is actually e-motion—energy in motion. Every emotion is a wave of chemical, physical, and physiological change in the body. Visualization becomes actualization when it moves electromagnetic energy through the body and creates neurophysiological changes.

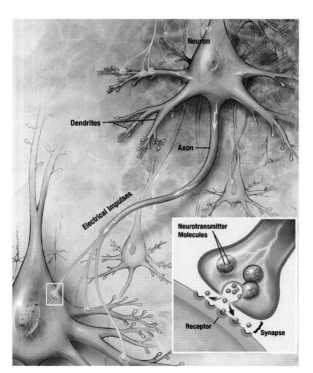

Figure 7.4. Visualization activates neurons in the brain, body, and skin that release neurochemicals that cause physiological changes.

THE GUT BRAIN, THE VAGUS NERVE, AND OUR EMOTIONAL HEALTH

In the past, dermatologists would often dismiss the idea that certain foods or emotional events affect the skin. And yet anyone who has sensitive skin knows that certain foods and emotions can definitely make the skin red, itchy, inflamed, and irritated. For example, those who suffer from acne will often discover that certain foods as well as stress can cause breakouts. Now science has confirmed that our gut and our brain talk to each other and influence each other, thereby affecting our emotions and energy.[2] In fact, all the organs talk to the brain all the time; however most people are not aware of this conversation. Understanding the brain-gut axis has become increasingly important in our understanding of how stress and emotions affect the body.

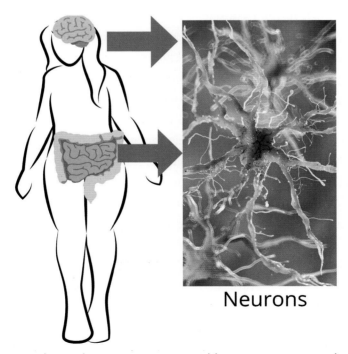

Neurons

Figure 7.7. The gut-brain axis is connected by neurotransmitters, hormones, and the vagus nerve.

In chapter 2 we noted that the enteric nervous system located in the intestines is a second brain, called the "gut brain." There are a number of factors that make the gut brain very important to our health and well-being. First, the enteric nervous system produces more than thirty neurotransmitters and has more neurons than the spine. Second, hormones and regulatory peptide molecules released from the gut brain can cross the brain barrier and influence a person's thinking and mood. And third, the large intestine is home to over 100,000 species of viruses and bacteria, which, as was recently discovered, can produce peptide regulators that affect the brain. With all their intelligence, humans are nevertheless controlled by their own microscopic inhabitants.[3]

The gut and the brain are connected through a very long nerve that wanders throughout the entire body. Because of its wandering nature, this nerve was named the *vagus nerve,* as in Latin *vagus* means "wandering" (hence the words *vague* and *vagabond,* which are derived from the same root). In the past, scientists mostly focused on the regulatory functions of the vagus nerve. They knew that it controls smooth muscle contraction and relaxation, the secretion of juices in the digestive tract, breathing, heartbeat, and some other body functions. What came as a total surprise, though, was the discovery that only 10 percent of all impulses traveling through the vagus nerve are regulatory impulses from the brain to the internal organs, while the other 90 percent are impulses that promptly carry information from the internal organs to the brain.[4]

Among its many tasks, the vagus nerve registers inflammation, levels of essential nutrients, the sensations in various organs, feelings of hunger, fullness, or satiation in the stomach, and energy metabolism. It is an essential energy pathway that sends an impressive amount of information from the organs to the brain.

After exiting the brain at the brain stem, the vagus nerve travels through the neck into the chest and abdomen. In the neck it regulates the muscles that control swallowing and speaking. Further down, in the chest, the vagus nerve controls the heart as a part of the parasympathetic nervous system. When the vagus activates, it slows down the heart rate. In the lungs, the vagus nerve relaxes and opens the bronchi-

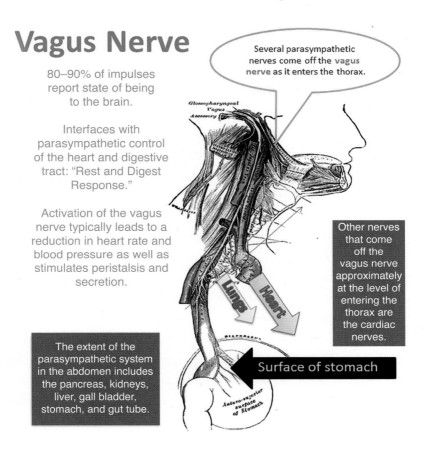

Vagus Nerve

80–90% of impulses report state of being to the brain.

Interfaces with parasympathetic control of the heart and digestive tract: "Rest and Digest Response."

Activation of the vagus nerve typically leads to a reduction in heart rate and blood pressure as well as stimulates peristalsis and secretion.

The extent of the parasympathetic system in the abdomen includes the pancreas, kidneys, liver, gall bladder, stomach, and gut tube.

Several parasympathetic nerves come off the **vagus nerve** as it enters the thorax.

Other nerves that come off the vagus nerve approximately at the level of entering the thorax are the cardiac nerves.

Surface of stomach

Figure 7.6. The vagus nerve wanders throughout the body.

oles. In the intestines it regulates digestion and intestinal movement. And as the vagus nerve wanders through each of the organs, regulating their activity, it collects sensory information from the gut and carries it to the brain, confirming the current scientific view that the gut, like the skin, is a large and important sensory organ.

It is because of the vagus nerve that the intestines can "taste" food much as the tongue does, and report the immediate effects as well as the more remote consequences of what it has consumed. The tongue can easily be fooled into accepting something as tasty despite the fact that it may have low nutritional value or is even toxic and damaging to the body. The gut sense is more attuned to the true needs of the body and provides more accurate information on the true health value of foods. Elevating one's body awareness and developing the habit of listening to the gut as we eat allows us to regulate our nutrition naturally.

The enteric nervous system records memories and remembers situations when a person experienced pain, injury, or extreme fear and discomfort. The gut brain can alert a person that something is not quite right and can do this much faster than the reasoning brain on the top of the spinal cord. Taoist practices of inner awareness allow us to fine-tune our intuition—very often called a "gut feeling"—to develop a new relationship with our food and own body sensations. Instead of using food to escape unpleasant feelings, we start to learn to discern between nuisance sensations and valuable information coming from the body's native intelligence. In this way, negative emotions can be processed and released, while food is reserved for supporting the body and enhancing the skin's radiance and beauty.

The vagus nerve also plays a major role in controlling inflammation. This is because being alive means eating food, and these days eating food usually means consuming allergens, pathogenic germs, and toxins. So the gut is always ready to ignite the defensive fire of inflammation by releasing and activating inflammatory chemicals. One of the functions of the vagus nerve is to curb this inflammation before it enters the bloodstream.

It has been demonstrated that excessive inflammation in the intestines can worsen symptoms of depression and anxiety through suppression of serotonin production. A 2013 study found that subjects who practiced what researchers described as a "loving kindness meditation" had better vagus nerve tone and experienced significant reduction in symptoms of anxiety and depression.[5] They proposed that the effect was mediated by both the enteric nervous system and the central nervous system. The perception of being loved, registered in the gut's nervous system, increased the activity of the vagus, and its signals in turn brought more calmness and peace to the brain. The Taoist version of a loving-kindness meditation is the Inner Smile practice, described in chapter 4, during which the practitioner sends the positive emotions of love, kindness, and compassion to their own organs.

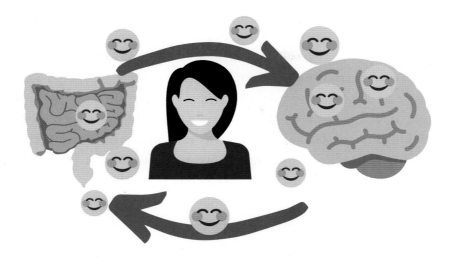

Figure 7.7. The cycle of comfort. A loving-kindness meditation sends signals of comfort to the gut brain, which in turn activates the vagus nerve, relaxing the body and reducing inflammation. The vagus nerve sends comforting signals to the brain, which stimulates relaxing thoughts, further enhancing the sense of comfort in the brain, which in turn sends more comfort signals back to the vagus nerve.

Another reason why it is important to do practices that activate a beneficial response from the vagus nerve involves our silent microscopic residents—the trillions of bacterial bodies that inhabit the gut. They are not just passive residents. Most people know that gut bacteria produce enzymes that break down food and help us digest fibers and certain nutrients. In addition, these bacteria produce sugars, fatty acids, and neurochemicals such as serotonin, and can stimulate the release of peptides and hormones from the gut, which then travel through the bloodstream to affect brain functions. Even though gut bacteria produce cytokines and regulatory peptides for their own needs, these substances also affect the brain and the nervous system.

The sensitive, receptive parts of the vagus nerve enter the gut mucosal layer and respond to the chemical signals of cytokines, nutrients, regulatory peptides, and hormones. Since gut microflora can secrete regulatory molecules, including serotonin, they can directly communicate with the vagus nerve and, through the vagus nerve, with the brain. Some gut bacteria signals such as the ones that are sent by the lactobacteria *Lactobacillus rhamnosus* are beneficial and produce calming and antianxiety effects, while others, such as those that are produced by the pathogenic microbe *Campylobacter jejuni*—one of the most common causes of food poisoning—elevate anxiety. Since the vagus nerve delivers information to the brain, it plays a major role in regulating the stress response. As studies of the vagus nerve and gut brain have revealed, many reactions traditionally viewed as purely psychological, such as stress,[6] depression,[7] and anxiety,[8] are closely linked to gut health and well-being. Inducing a relaxation response activates the vagus nerve, curbs inflammation, and ensures the production of beneficial regulatory molecules and neurochemicals.

BEAUTY SLEEP AND EMOTIONAL DETOX

Many people feel uncomfortable if they don't get a chance to brush their teeth before going to sleep because they can practically feel all the food they've eaten stuck in their teeth, causing decay. Since people need to eat, they cannot expect their teeth to remain perfectly clean all day long. The same is true for negative emotions. It is impossible to avoid being triggered or inconvenienced by life. The key is to make sure that the negative emotions that arise are cleared and released from the body to ensure they do not get stuck, causing lasting damage.

Taoists maintain that when all the organs get overwhelmed with negative emotional energy they dump it into the skin. This is why cleansing the body of negative emotional energies is essential to creating inner beauty and outer radiance. Emotional detox has to go hand-in-hand with physical detox. While sleeping, we are resting and rejuvenating the organs that remove toxins from the blood and body, which is why we are admonished to get our "beauty sleep."

Science now confirms that the skin is an important detoxing organ that removes toxins through sweating and oil production. When the blood is "dirty" with metabolic toxins, the skin has to work extra hard to detox the body. Toxic emotional energy deposited in the organs and spilling over into the skin creates unhealthy conditions, diminishing the skin's radiance and its ability to regenerate. Chronic stress and undigested emotions upset the gut brain, with all its trillions of powerful microscopic residents. The vagus nerve detects the discomfort and inflammation and sends more alarm signals to the brain. The brain in turn is flooded with unpleasant, anxious, upsetting thoughts, which disturb sleep. The next morning, the brain and the body are tired, the gut is heavy and upset, food has not been properly digested, and the kidneys and liver have to work extra hard to remove toxins. The result is a dull complexion, hollow circles under the eyes, and other skin issues. Taoist practices of emotional detox, when used along with good sleep hygiene, can help us release negative emotions and restore the skin's radiance and beauty.

It is important to have the very last meal for the day at least four to five hours before going to sleep. Taoist masters actually recommend leaving at least eight hours from the last meal of the day and sleep, but if this seems too extreme, at least four hours is better than eating right before trying to go to sleep. As well, the evening meal should be a light meal. The Tao says, "In the morning, eat like a king. During lunch, eat like a prince. During diner, eat like a beggar." They did not mean eat like a beggar who suddenly got a place at the king's table, but a "beggar" who eats very little as a matter of course. It is important to make meals as healthy and toxin-free as possible, and to avoid alcohol and too much sugar, particularly at the last meal of the day. During sleep, when the body is relaxed and we aren't expending energy on moving, speaking, eating, or working, the body cleanses itself from damaged proteins, sick and damaged cells (including cancerous cells), chemical toxins and pollutants, and, of course, toxic emotional energy. When we eat right before sleep, we have to digest the food we ate, and this takes approximately four hours. When most of the food is digested, the liver filters the blood, and its cells attach a chemical compound called *urea* to all the toxins that need to be eliminated. Then these urea-marked toxins are detected by the kidneys and properly removed. With late-night meals, however, the body has much less time to detox, and the result is that toxins accumulate, and this is reflected in the skin.

It is important that the room you sleep in is dark, because darkness during the night switches the metabolism over to melatonin production. Melatonin is a hormone produced by the pineal gland. Its production increases when it is dark, and it puts the body into a more relaxed and restful state. Also, melatonin is an important antioxidant that helps the skin look younger. If at all possible try to sleep in a room without running computers or other electronic devices. The room should be peaceful and comfortable. The Tao advises at least seven hours of sleep to keep the brain healthy and vibrant. It is also recommended that we go to sleep between 10 and 11 p.m. to allow the liver to work on toxins. During sleep, the brain clears out the proteins that cause neurodegenerative conditions such as Alzheimer's.[9] In the morning, Taoist practitioners drink a glass of pure, clean water (not tea or coffee) to flush toxins out of the kidneys.

SIX HEALING SOUNDS MEDITATION FOR EMOTIONAL DETOX

The Six Healing Sounds meditation helps remove toxic emotional energy as well as excess CO_2. It is a beautiful ritual that includes, slow, mindful breathing, visualization of the organs, stretching, and, of course, the six sounds that correspond to the organs. When done before sleep, at the end of a busy or emotional day, it creates a wonderful state of relaxation and calm that will lead to a beautiful, deep, restful sleep. Once the steps are memorized it is not always necessary to go through every organ. If there is no time or you are very tired, you can work with the specific emotions that caused problems during the day. If someone made you angry, it's important to release that anger. If you felt sad, it's important to release that sadness. If you felt worried, focus on worry and then release it. Never go to sleep with negative energy stuck in the organs, because it will negatively affect the entire body, including the skin, not to mention disrupt one's sleep.

All the sounds are barely audible and produced on a long, slow exhalation at the level of a whisper.

Six Healing Sounds and Their Organ Locations

1. **Lungs (*sssssss*):** To produce this sound, inhale, smile slightly, put your tongue behind the teeth and let the hissing sound of *sssssss* emerge on a long exhale with little effort. It is not a loud sound, but rather a quiet, snakelike hiss. The lung sound clears negative emotions of grief and sadness.

2. **Kidneys (*chooooo*):** Inhale, round your lips, and then exhale, making a *ch* sound as in *choice* and *chi,* and an *oo* sound as in *choose.* The kidney sound clears negative emotions related to fear.

3. **Liver (*shhhhhh*):** Inhale and slowly exhale, producing the sound *shhhhhh,* as if you wanted to hush someone. The liver sound clears negative emotions of anger, resentment, jealousy, and greed.

4. **Heart (*haaaaw*):** Inhale, then open and round your lips, forming the sound of *h* as in *heart,* then continue on a long exhalation as if with a sigh of relief, *aaaw.* The heart sound clears the negative emotions of arrogance, harshness, hatred, cruelty, rage, impatience.

5. **Spleen (*whooooo*):** Inhale, form the sound of the letter *w,* and proceed with the sound *whooo,* like an owl, produced on a long, slow exhalation. The spleen sound clears negative emotions of worry, doubt, and mistrust.

6. **Triple Warmer (*heeeeee*):** Inhale, form the sound of the letter *h,* then release an *eeee* sound on a long, slow exhalation, as in *leap* or *heap.* The triple warmer sound balances the temperature of the Upper Warmer (the area above the diaphragm, which often gets very hot due to more intense metabolic activity), Middle Warmer (the area between the diaphragm and the navel, where the digestive organs are located and which often has slower metabolism especially if a person is leading a sedentary lifestyle), and Lower Warmer (reproductive organs and organs responsible for elimination of waste, which often get too cold and need warming up). The sound and corresponding movement (p. 139) helps to distribute heat evenly throughout the body. This sound is different from other sounds because it is not connected to any particular emotion, color, or element.

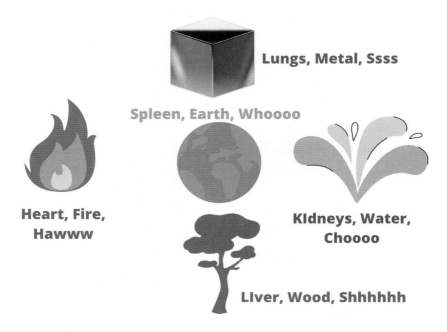

Lungs, Metal, Ssss

Spleen, Earth, Whoooo

Heart, Fire, Hawww

Kidneys, Water, Choooo

Liver, Wood, Shhhhhh

Figure 7.8. Five of the six healing sounds. The triple warmer is not shown because it is a balancing and finishing sound and as such is not associated with any element or color. The sound of the triple warmer is *heeeeee*.

Six Healing Sounds Chi Kung

Lungs

Element: metal
Color: white
Sound: *sssssss*
Positive energies: courage, justice, righteousness
Negative energies: grief, sadness, depression

1. Sit straight on the edge of a chair. Plant both feet on the floor. Imagine your feet are growing roots and connecting you to the earth.
2. Take a deep breath and slowly let it out. Relax.
3. Gently rock your spine side to side, starting from the base of your spine and gradually progressing to rocking the neck area. Imagine

you have a tail growing from your tailbone down into the ground. As you rock your spine, imagine a fiery dragon swimming up your spine, enlivening and energizing it.

4. Think of a person you love or imagine a source of loving energy in front of you. When you start feeling that love, smile. Imagine your smile as being sunshine warming the surface of a lake. Smile with this smile. Take a deep inhalation and exhale. Relax.

5. Bring your attention to your lungs. Smile into your lungs. See your lungs filling with white light. Place your hands near your lungs, palms facing the lungs. Feel their energy.

6. For each lung, look deeply inside the lung and move your eyes left and right, back and forth, imagining sweeping the inside of each lung with your inner eyes, while moving your hands together with your eyes left and right, back and forth. Do this back-and-forth movement of the eyes and hands thirty-six times. Think of all the feelings that can collapse your lungs, impede breathing, and deflate you. Imagine gathering them up as cloudy, gray colors. (Note: For each organ, the eyes are physically moved side-to-side and at the same time they are visualized moving inside the organ. Such repetitive lateral movement of the eyes has been shown to neurologically reset the emotional state and is now used in many therapies such as Eye Movement Desensitization and Reprocessing (EMDR). The difference is that in the Taoist practices physical eye movement is combined with movement of the hands *and* visualization of eyes moving *inside* the organ.)

7. Slowly begin to inhale as you gracefully raise your hands to the level of your chest with the fingers of both hands pointing toward each other. Then turn palms upward with fingers on both hands still pointing toward each other. Continue raising them until your arms are stretched with your elbows slightly bent and your palms are above your head, with palms upward (fig. 7.9). Look at the back of your palms, smile, and begin a long and slow exhale. As you slowly lower your hands imagine releasing a cloud of foggy, cloudy energy with the sound *sssssss*. Guide this energy down to the ground with

your eyes and your hands. You can add the mantra, "Forgive and forget. Release, relax, and let it go."

8. Next, assume a resting position. This position is the same between each sound. Place your hands on your knees. Imagine negative energy leaving your body and going down into the earth to be composted.

9. Next you are going to clear your brain. Raise your hands to your forehead with your palms toward your forehead. Smile, look up into your brain, and move your eyes and hands left and right in a lateral motion while imagining your eyes moving *inside* your brain. Move your hands and your eyes left and right thirty-six times, clearing all memories of sadness, grief, and depression out of your brain. This part will be repeated for each organ and each sound. After you have finished clearing the brain, proceed with the lung sound once again as described above, finishing with guiding the foggy, gray, and cloudy energy down to the ground.

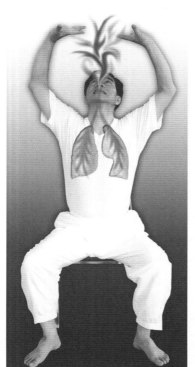

Figure 7.9. Position for healing sounds of the lungs.

10. Place your hands near your lungs, palms facing them, and visualize sending vibrant white energy of courage, fairness, righteousness, and the metal element into your lungs. Imagine white light radiating into your skin and large intestine.

Kidneys

Element: water
Color: blue
Sound: *chooooo*
Positive energies: stillness, tranquility, gentleness
Negative energies: fear (often as a result of shock or trauma)

1. Bring your attention to your kidneys. Become aware of the energy of the kidneys. Smile into your kidneys. Fill your kidneys with deep blue light and the element of water.

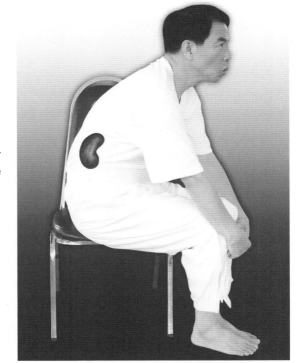

Figure 7.10. Position for healing sounds of the kidneys.

2. Rub your hands together to make them warm and hold your hands next to the kidney area on the back, palms facing your back. Look to the left and the right into each of your kidneys, and repeat this lateral eye and hands movement thirty-six times. Imagine you are looking for dark, cloudy, gray colors and the cold energy of fear. As you exhale, lean forward, hug your knees with both hands, and slowly exhale, producing the sound *chooooo* while looking forward (fig. 7.10). Imagine guiding any dark, cloudy, gray colors down into the ground with your eyes. Repeat the mantra, "Forgive and forget. Release, relax, and let go."

3. Place your hands on your knees for a resting position. Imagine negative energy of fear leaving your body and returning to the earth.

4. Clear the negative energy from your brain, as described above, and then proceed with guiding this energy to the ground this time with the kidney sound *chooooo*. You can repeat the mantra, "Forgive and forget. Release, relax, and let it go."

5. Hold your palms on your back, next to your kidneys, and send blue light, calmness, tranquility, and gentleness into your kidneys.

Liver

Element: wood
Color: green
Sound: *shhhhhh*
Positive energies: kindness, forgiveness, generosity
Negative energies: greed, jealousy, anger, guilt

1. Bring your attention to your liver. Smile into your liver. Become aware of the energy of the liver, the color green, and the wood element.

2. Look left and right into your liver thirty-six times while holding your palms next to your liver, with palms facing the liver. Move your palms and your eyes together, gathering negative energy. Imagine you are seeing greed, jealousy, anger, and guilt as dark, cloudy, gray colors.

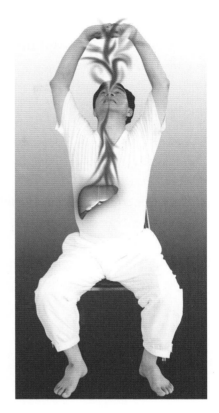

Figure 7.11. Position for healing
sounds of the liver.

3. Slowly inhale as you lift your arms up as you did for the lung sound. This time, interlace your fingers as you turn your palms upward. Instead of raising your arms straight up, lean to the left, creating a slight tension and a feeling of openness in the liver. Look up into the backs of your hands, and slowly exhale the sound *shhhhhh*. As you lower your hands toward the ground, imagine sending dark, cloudy, gray colors down into the ground. Repeat the mantra, "Forgive and forget. Release, relax, and let go."

4. Do the clearing of emotional energy in the brain using the same process as described above, but with the liver sound.

5. Finish the liver clearing by holding your hands on your liver area, palms facing inward, smiling loving sunshine into your liver, filling it with the clean, clear, pure green light of kindness and generosity and the element of wood. Feel good in your liver. Smile deeper into your liver.

6. Rest and imagine your liver filling with the warm green light of
   the wood element. Feel the nourishing, strong, generous energy of
   wood in your liver.

❷ Heart

Element: fire
Color: red
Sound: *haaaaw*
Positive energies: love, joy, patience, happiness
Negative energies: hatred, arrogance, indifference, rage, cruelty

1. Bring your attention to your heart. Hold your hands palms facing the heart. Feel the energy of the heart. Smile into your heart.

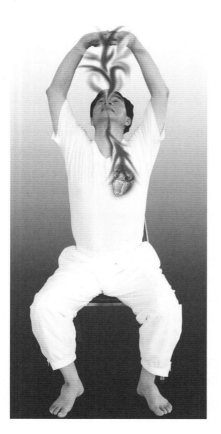

Figure 7.12. Position for healing
sounds of the heart.

Imagine connecting with the warm red light of love, joy, and happiness in your heart and the element of fire.

2. Look left and right into your heart while moving your hands and your eyes laterally. Imagine moving your eyes inside your heart thirty-six times, looking for the dark negative energies of rage, hate, cruelty, impatience, or arrogance.

3. Inhale and exhale slowly with the sound *haaaaaw* as you raise your arms above your head, interlace your fingers, and turn your palms upward. Lean to the right, feeling the openness in your heart. Guide any dark, cloudy, gray colors down into the ground. Repeat the mantra, "Forgive and forget. Release, relax and let it go."

4. Return to the resting position. Place your hands on your knees. Rock your spine back and forth. Imagine any negative energy going down into the ground.

5. Do the clearing of emotional energy in the brain using the brain-clearing process described for other organs, but use the heart sound, *haaaaw*.

6. Replenish the energy of your heart by smiling into your heart and sending it the warm red light of love, happiness, gratitude, and joy.

Spleen

Element: earth
Color: yellow
Sound: *whooooo*
Positive energies: trust, confidence, fairness, openness, faith
Negative energies: mistrust, imbalance, anxiety, worry

1. Bring your attention to your spleen. Become aware of the energy of your spleen. Hold your palms facing your spleen. Smile into your spleen. Fill your spleen with yellow light, confidence, trust, and faith, and the element of earth.

2. Move your hands and your eyes in the lateral motion, while imagining your eyes looking left and right inside your spleen thirty-six times, imagining you are gathering the dark, heavy, gray, cloudy energy of doubt, mistrust, and worry.

3. The movement for this organ is different. This time, exhale the sound *whooooo* while leaning forward and gently pressing your left side under your rib cage with both hands, releasing dark, cloudy, gray colors and guiding them down into the ground. Imagine sending negative energy down to the ground. Repeat the mantra, "Forgive and forget. Release, relax, and let it go."

4. Place your hands on your lap, rocking your spine back and forth, releasing any dark and cloudy energy down into the ground.

5. Do the clearing of emotional energy in the brain using the same brain-clearing process as for other organs, but use the spleen sound, *whooooo*.

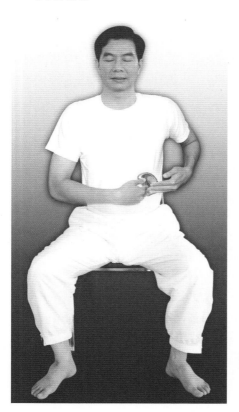

Figure 7.13. Position for healing sounds of the spleen.

6. Hold your palms near your spleen and imagine the stable, secure, supportive, and fertile energy of earth in your spleen. Imagine the earth taking all your worries away from you.

☯ Triple Warmer

Note: The Triple Warmer is a meridian that involves the thyroid, thymus, and adrenal glands and controls the fight-flight-freeze response.

Element: no element; it is a finishing and balancing sound
Color: no color; it is a finishing and balancing sound
Sound: *heeeeee*

1. Lie down or lean back comfortably in a chair.
2. Raise your arms overhead.
3. Inhale, and then as you exhale, whisper a long *heeeeee* while slowly sweeping your hands over your body from your crown downward.

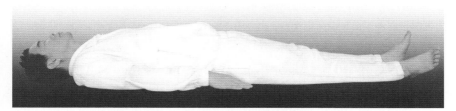

Figure 7.14. Position for healing sounds of the triple warmer.

4. Repeat three times.
5. This is a balancing and finishing step. At this point all organs are cleared and filled with vibrant energy.

☯ Beauty Chi Kung Emotional Detox

The following exercise uses the six healing sounds to help you release the stress or emotional upsets of your day.

1. Sit straight on the edge of a chair. Take a deep breath and shake your spine. Plant your feet on the floor and imagine deep roots growing from the soles of your feet into the ground. Become aware of your Bubbling Springs points; these are the soft spots below the toes (see chapter 8, figure 8.10, for an illustration of this point). Breathe through the Bubbling Springs, inhaling golden light from the earth. Smile into your body.

2. Think of your morning, for example, between the hours of 8 a.m. and 10 a.m. Check if there are any negative emotions that may still be stuck in your body. For example, you read an upsetting news story and got angry. Work on your liver and release the anger with the sound *shhhhhh*. If you received sad news and still feel sadness in your body, work on your lungs and release the sadness with the sound *sssssss*. You can spend more time on this particular emotion, making sure it is released.

3. Think of your late morning, such as between 10 a.m. and noon. Were there any emotions that came up then that you still feel in your body? Notice the emotion and release it using the sound that corresponds to that emotion.

4. Repeat the same process with the time intervals noon to 2 p.m.; 2 p.m. to 4 p.m.; 4 p.m. to 6 p.m.; 6 p.m. to 8 p.m.; and 8 p.m. to 10 p.m. With practice, such a review can be done quickly, so that eventually you won't have as many negative emotions cropping up during the day, and there won't be a need for such a detailed practice.

5. Always finish with the Triple Warmer sound *heeeeee* to balance your energy. Remember to smile.

This practice will help the organs feel cleaner and lighter. Eventually, all built-up negative emotions will be released, and the overall level of stress and unhappiness will go down. You will experience deeper and more restful sleep, which is essential for body and skin regeneration and replenishment; a softer and more radiant glow, which will make the skin look younger and more beautiful; better digestion and absorption of nutrients, which will help your skin repair and rebuild itself; and overall a more relaxed and friendly expression and a stable mood and temperament, which will improve your work, relationships, and overall health.

What we can vividly imagine becomes real to the body. When you start using your imagination intentionally, you activate your natural gift of creation. To make this practice really work as it should, it is important to know the locations and shapes of the organs. Once you visualize an organ, the brain region associated with this organ activates and sends signals to that part of the nervous system that rules that particular organ. When the nervous system of the organ activates, it releases neurochemicals, depending on the emotion. Images of relaxation and positive emotions relax the body and create pleasant, warm sensations. The gut affects the brain through the vagus nerve as described in this chapter. The Six Healing Sounds meditation activates the vagus, sending signals of peace and love to the brain. It releases stress and allows the body and skin to repair and regenerate. It is extremely important to release negative emotions every evening. This will ensure a deeper, more restful sleep and allow the skin to heal, renew, and regenerate every night, emerging more radiant and beautiful every morning.

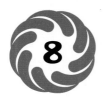

Preserving Youthful Beauty with the Microcosmic Orbit

> *Beauty is a form of Genius; it is higher, indeed, than Genius, as it needs no explanation. It is one of the great facts of the world, like sunlight.*
>
> OSCAR WILDE, *THE PICTURE OF DORIAN GRAY*

The nineteenth-century British writer Oscar Wilde wrote the provocative novel *The Picture of Dorian Gray,* in which he tells the story of a young man gifted with exquisite beauty who made a careless and dangerous wish. He wanted his portrait to bear all the consequences of aging so that his own face could remain as young and beautiful as on the day the portrait was painted. Soon he realizes that every time he gives in to his dark passions and temptations, his face remains fresh, innocent, and beautiful, but the portrait changes and starts looking less beautiful and less innocent. At first, Dorian is very happy that he can do whatever he wishes, because his beautiful and innocent face protects him from accusations. But in the end, the portrait acquires so many hideous features and becomes so repulsively ugly that Dorian Gray cannot bear looking at it or even having it in his possession. He kills his portrait, and with it, himself. The truth of this story, which Wilde reveals so brilliantly, is that skin is a truth-teller. And the older we are, the more revealing our skin becomes. Many people spend a lot of money and energy trying to preserve their youth and beauty.* However not many people realize that the skin reveals more than just one's age; it also reveals the hidden negative emotions we hold and our current state of health and well-being.

In the past, people had no choice but to live in the skin they were born with. Today there is an impressive array of available skin-care products: cosmetic injections, plastic surgery, laser treatments, chemical peels, dermabrasion, and other means to erase wrinkles, remove undereye bags and dark circles, tighten up the face, polish and plump lips and cheeks, and remove blemishes. These methods can help you achieve a more youthful and well-groomed complexion, but they cannot hide a lack of vitality or conceal excessive grumpiness, bitterness, resentment, anger, and other negative emotions, which tend to accumulate as we age. We look younger and more beautiful when we have luminous, vibrant, radiant energy flowing throughout our body, and older and less attractive when we are depleted, exhausted, and drained. A body that is filled with positive, loving, smiling energy looks and feels better compared to a body twisted in angry knots. Most people know that their negative emotions, stress, and physical depletion make them look less attractive, so they try to build a wall around their heart to hide their personal energy. Practically everybody knows how to put on a mask to have a better chance at being accepted, but this requires that we hold tension in the body, and the older we get, the more energy we need to expend to keep all those negative emotions safely locked away in the body.

---

*In the article "How Much Do Americans Spend on Their Looks Each Year," published in *Cosmetics and Toiletries* (December 14, 2022), it is noted that women spend more than men do on their looks, that the average American spends $630 on cosmetic procedures, and that nearly one in six Americans spend more on beauty and wellness than they can afford.

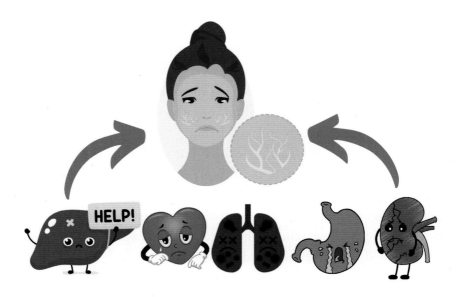

Figure 8.1. Negative emotions held in the body show up
on the face and the skin.

The skin is connected to every other organ in the body and interacts with the immune, endocrine, and nervous systems. They all share the same chemical messengers and influence one another's functions. Nowadays many scientists propose that rather than study the nervous, immune, and endocrine systems of the skin separately, we should consider discussing the psycho-neuro-immune-endocrine function of the skin.[1]

For example, the skin plays a pivotal role in the stress response. If we experience pain or discomfort on our skin, our brain's alarm system gets activated. In the same way, if a scary or alarming thought flashes through your mind, the skin immediately receives an alert and starts activating its immune defense mechanisms. If you're a chronic worrier, your skin's immune system will become exhausted and start overreacting, resulting in rashes, irritations, and allergies.[2] Many skin conditions such as eczema and psoriasis have been linked to chronic stress.[3]

Science confirms that mindfulness, Tai Chi, yoga, and breath-based meditation can reduce chronic inflammation and help prevent diseases caused by chronic stress.[4]

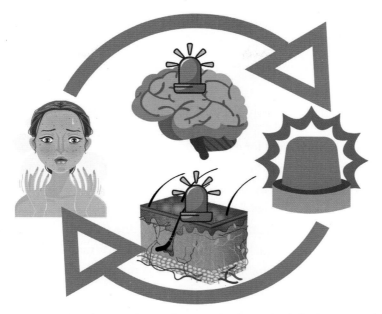

Figure 8.2. The skin sends an alarm to the brain and the brain sends an alarm back to the skin, creating a vicious cycle of stress.

Our thoughts and emotions affect our biochemistry, electrophysiology, physiology, and even our genes. A rapidly growing branch of modern science, epigenetics, reveals to us that our genes change their activities throughout our life. Certain foods, physical activities (such as aerobic exercise), hypnosis, and meditation have been shown to alter gene activity, switching protein synthesis to a younger state. Today there is enough scientific evidence to show that relaxation, breathing, and visualization can reduce inflammation and distress in the skin.[5] A 2008 study used a DNA microarray to evaluate gene activity before and after a hypnotic experience. The analysis revealed that hypnosis activated genes associated with (1) heightened activity of stem cells, (2) a reduction in cellular oxidative stress, and (3) a reduction in chronic inflammation.[6] Another study evaluated the physiological effects of slow, intentional breathing. The researchers concluded that such breathing techniques can improve overall health through heightened interoception, which is defined as the sense of the internal state of the body, which can be both conscious and unconscious.[7]

Of course, Taoist masters discovered thousands of years ago that taking control of the inner sense of the body opens possibilities for improving the regulation of the body's systems.

ENERGY HIGHWAYS IN THE BODY

Taoist masters discovered long ago that it is possible to learn how to sense the movement of chi in the body and use this sense of interoception to improve and direct energy flow throughout the body. They found that energy in the body follows certain paths or channels, as is well-known by practitioners of Traditional Chinese Medicine (TCM). Though the complete system of channels is quite complex, Taoist masters found that there are certain major channels that serve as the main energy highways that connect the body's energetic pathways, and when these major channels are blocked, it greatly affects one's vitality and health. So we don't need to study the complexities of TCM and learn the locations of all the various meridians to learn how to take care of the major energy channels, as Taoist practices are quite efficient at unblocking these channels to create a stronger and better energy flow throughout the entire body.

This is easiest to understand by picturing a busy city with many streets. It may take a long time to get from one end of the city to another by using only surface streets, but it is much faster to get around by using the highway that encircles the city. A major accident blocking that highway will slow traffic down throughout the city. The same way, energy blockages in the major energy channels blocks all the other channels and diminishes one's overall vitality and radiance.

To release negative emotions in the body, we use the Six Healing Sounds meditation described in chapter 7, and to replenish the energy of the organs, we use Inner Smile Chi Kung, described in chapter 4. These practices, which allow energy to flow through the body unimpeded, ensure that the skin has enough life force to regenerate and renew. But if the major highway is blocked, it will be much more difficult to release negative energy and replenish the organs. Therefore, to achieve vitality and true beauty, it is important to know how to open the major energy channels in the body.

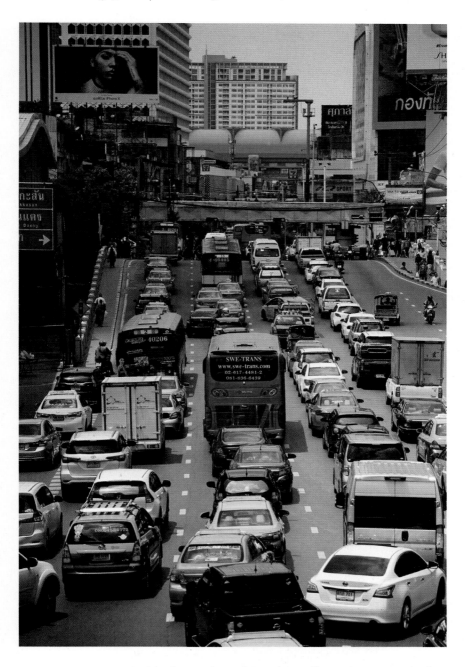

Figure 8.3. A jammed highway slows down the traffic in the entire city the same way that a blockage in one of the major channels blocks the flow of chi in the body.

It's like a dam blocking a mighty river. If the dam breaks, water flows everywhere, causing destruction and devastation. If, however, there is a system of channels, and they are all open, water can easily flow through them, and this will prevent any damage. The same is true for the body and the emotions. When the body has a well-developed and open system of channels, it can safely deal with even very strong and powerful emotions. In Taoist practice it is believed that even negative emotions can be transformed back into the life force to replenish the body. This requires having an efficient system that can easily move energy.

The sensation of chi in the body is very individual; it may be felt as warmth, movement, buzzing, tingling, or other sensations. Many people do not feel anything at all at first, as it takes time to develop the ability to sense energy. One important thing to realize is that this energy is quite real. The life force flows through every organ, including the skin, because this is what keeps us alive. As chi flows, it also activates the flow of blood, lymph, regulatory molecules, oxygen, and trophic factors that are critical to cellular maintenance and regeneration. Using the Taoist method of inner sensing, it is possible to learn how to maintain a healthy and vibrant energy flow through the body's major energy highways, to replenish the vital organs, release negative energy, and ensure that the skin, our largest organ, has enough life force to renew, regenerate, and be beautiful.

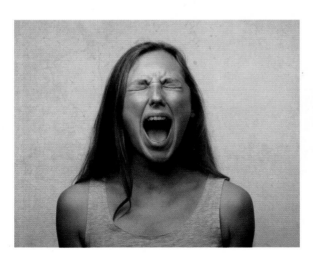

Figure 8.4. Negative emotions, if not released, can take over the entire body.

THE MAJOR ENERGY CENTERS

The body's major energy centers have a high density of blood vessels, nerve fibers, lymph vessels, and endocrine glands that store, receive, and transform energy. Taoists of the past did not know modern anatomy, physics, biochemistry, or neurology, yet they were the first to discover that electrical energy needs a closed circuit in which to flow. In a house, if there is there a break in the electrical wiring, the whole house will go dark unless it has an independent electrical circuit to safeguard against power outages. Fortunately, the body is designed with such safeguards in place. If electricity is blocked in one area, the body knows how to reroute the current. Yet to properly nourish the entire body, it is important to ensure that the river of gold that is our chi flows through every organ, every tissue, and every cell. Some of our organs seem to be capable of generating and storing more energy than others and can serve as batteries or reservoirs of energy. These are the brain, the heart, the intestines, the kidneys, and the sexual organs (both male and female), all of which store mitochondria, the cellular generators of electricity.

Chi Storage Centers in the Body

- **Brain, or Upper Tan Tien:** The brain consumes energy at a very high rate. Even in a resting state the brain can consume 20 percent of the body's total oxygen (burning it and producing CO_2 and energy). The brain can overheat if it works intensely without adequate movement of energy throughout the rest of the body. Its major endocrine glands, the pineal and the pituitary, regulate the functions of the entire body. The pineal gland is a small, pinecone-shaped structure located in the deep center of the brain, approximately on the same level as the third eye. It protrudes from hypothalamus and produces melatonin, a hormone that is secreted in response to light that regulates circadian rhythms. Melatonin is also connected to the regulation of the reproductive organs. The pituitary gland, a pea-sized gland located at the base of the brain, approximately on the same level as the mideyebrow point, or third eye, is considered the master gland because it controls other hormones, producing prolactin, adrenocorticotropic (ACTH) and growth hormones (released during stress), thyroid-stimulating hormone, and oxytocin (the love and bonding hormone, which in breastfeeding women stimulates lactation).

- **Heart center, or Middle Tan Tien:** The heart produces a lot of energy because its cells are packed with the cellular power stations that are the mitochondria. The heart is a very active organ that requires a lot of energy, as myocardial mitochondria must have an abundant oxygen supply to provide enough energy for the heart muscle to work optimally. If the oxygen supply decreases, such as when the blood vessels develop atherosclerotic plaques, the heart muscle suffers, and this leads to cardiac disease. The heart cannot store energy and is not a good battery. In Taoist tradition it is believed that the heart can connect to other people and to the entire universe through the energy of unconditional love. The heart generates a powerful electromagnetic field that can be felt by other people. According to the HeartMath Institute, the magnetic field produced by the heart can extend up to three feet from the body and is more than a hundred times greater in strength than the brain's magnetic field.

- **Solar plexus:** The solar plexus is a hub of nerve fibers radiating in all directions and controlling organs in the abdominal cavity. It is a part of the sympathetic nervous system and can orchestrate the fight-or-flight response.

- **Navel center, or Lower Tan Tien:** The Lower Tan Tien is located below the navel. In the Taoist tradition it is considered our main energy storage center, or biobattery. This is the enteric nervous system, which is part of the autonomic nervous system and is sometimes called the "second brain." As we now know, this "brain" plays an essential role in regulating the body's functions. It's a rich source of neurochemicals that affect mood and well-being. Recently scientists discovered a new organ in the abdominal cavity—a fold of connective tissue containing nerve tissue, blood vessels, and lymph vessels that serves as a biocomputer, regulating the functions of all the abdominal organs. This is the mesentery, which is now considered a major organ of the enteric nervous system.[8]

- **Sexual energy center, or the Ovarian/Sperm Palace:** The sexual center is located in the pelvic area and contains the nerve plexus that controls the sexual organs and other organs in the pelvic area. The Sexual Center is not a physical organ. It corresponds to the nervous and circulation connections in this area related to the sexual organs.

- **Perineum, or the Gate of Life and Death:** Taoists believe that people can leak energy from the Gate of Life and Death. They also say that we can train the perineum and turn it into a chi muscle that can pull energy into the anus and into the channels through the body all the way to the brain.

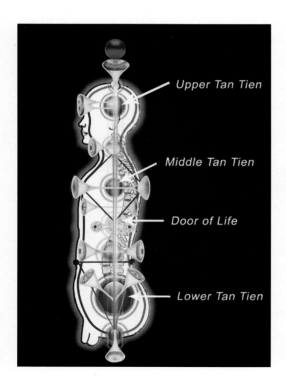

Figure 8.5. The major energy centers and their locations.

COMBINING THREE FIRES INTO ONE

In addition to their physiological roles, the organs, as we know, also have energetic roles. The Upper Tan Tien, Middle Tan Tien, and Lower Tan Tien are the major energetic "fires." The Upper Tan Tien, or brain, cannot store too much energy because it can easily overheat. Modern life causes people to focus outwardly and consume too much negative information, which generates a lot of heat in the brain, creating conditions for mental imbalance. However this center can also be used to connect to the vast energy available in the universe. The Middle Tan Tien, or Heart, also cannot store too much energy because it too easily overheats. It is better used to multiply one's emotional energy and radiate it out to connect to other people. Taoists maintain that the heart is connected to the unconditional love available throughout the universe. It is the Lower Tan Tien, or the abdominal center, that serves as the body's main biobattery; it stores large amounts of energy to supply the body's needs.

Since the skin is closely connected to the brain, anything that affects the brain will affect the skin. Worry, anxiety, anger, or resentment, which overheat the brain, will cause skin problems such as rashes, red blotches, swelling, and so forth. When negative energy gets stuck in the heart, it causes overheating and overwhelm, blocking the heart's radiance. Because the heart cannot hold too much heat, it will dump any negative emotional energy into the solar plexus, which affects breathing. When the heart is overwhelmed with negative emotions such as grudges, resentment, and impatience, the skin is inevitably affected.

When the brain, heart, and gut are disconnected and have forgotten how to work together, the person will have to wrestle with their inner conflicts and will often feel out of control in their life. In such situations the person will fight with their partner, shout at their children, eat food they know is unhealthy, and give in to the temptations of shopping, alcohol consumption, excessive TV watching, or sexual desires. All these behaviors are symptoms of the body's efforts to relieve the pressure of imbalanced energies. Since we do not have a portrait like Dorian Gray's hidden in the attic, all these dark passions are going to leave their expressions on our skin. Taoist practice teaches us that it is very important to bring excess heat down from the brain and heart, to the Lower Tan Tien. This means we must have a clear understanding of the location of the three major fires and know how to use the mind/ heart/eye power to bring the excess heat down.

The Three Fires

- The Upper Tan Tien fire is located in the center of the brain. It can be found by drawing an imaginary line first from the third eye to the back of the skull, then drawing another imaginary line connecting the tips of the ears, and finally drawing a line from the crown down to the perineum (fig. 8.6, p. 154).
- The Middle Tan Tien, or heart fire, can be located by drawing a line first from a point located one inch above the tip of the sternum on the midline, to thoracic vertebra number 5 (T5), and then finding its intersection with the line that goes from the crown to the perineum.
- The Lower Tan Tien fire can be located by drawing an imaginary line from the navel to the Door of Life, which is the point on the spine opposite the navel, found between lumbar vertebras 2 and 3 (L2 and L3). The fire is located below the intersection, in a triangular space between the navel, the Door of Life (i.e., the kidney center), and the sexual center (fig. 8.7, p. 154).

To combine all three fires together, focus on the center of the brain first. Then imagine spiraling all the thoughts and all the energy down to the heart center, and continue spiraling further down to the Lower Tan Tien so that the mind can rest and replenish its energy. This mental exercise will quickly create a more balanced, centered, and calm feeling.

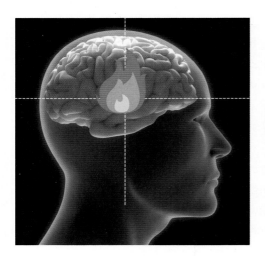

Figure 8.6.
The Upper Tan Tien fire.

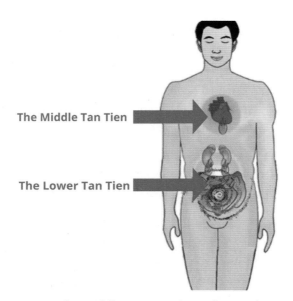

Figure 8.7. The Middle Tan Tien (heart fire) and Lower Tan Tien
(abdominal fire).

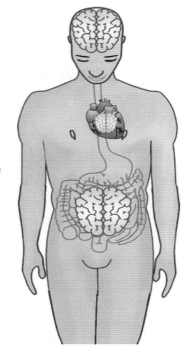

Figure 8.8.
Combining the three
fires into one.

THE MICROCOSMIC ORBIT

Taoist masters say there are two major energy highways that together follow a path around the body; they call this the Microcosmic Orbit. The first channel is the yang channel, which is the governor channel. It starts at the perineum, flows through the tailbone, inside the sacrum, up the spinal cord under the skin, under the skull to the crown, and then down the skull to the third eye and mideyebrow, through the sinuses, to the hard palate.

The other channel is the yin channel, which is also called the functional or conception channel. It starts at the perineum, goes up under the skin, following the midline through the navel, solar plexus, heart center, throat center, and to the lower jaw. The two channels become one closed circuit, or orbit, when the tongue is lifted and pressed to the upper palate. Using mind, eye, and heart power we can direct the flow of energy through this orbit, which distributes chi from the major energy centers throughout the body, preventing excesses and blockages. As a result, the skin develops radiance, the posture becomes more upright and confident, and the body feels vital, vibrant, and youthful. The Microcosmic Orbit unites the body as an integrated whole, with mind, body, and spirit flowing together to elevate the life force.

The Main Points of the Microcosmic Orbit

1. **Navel:** The Microcosmic Orbit starts and ends at the navel center, located 1.5 inches below the navel. The navel is our first connection to the outside world from which we received nutrition and oxygen while in utero. This area retains its energetic significance throughout life. The navel is the point for centering and connection to all the organs. It is also the entrance to the Lower Tan Tien cauldron, which is the place where we gather, transform, and store energy. The navel area can store large amounts of chi and can process and balance energy. When the navel center is open and balanced, it is reflected in more centered and balanced behavior. When the navel is blocked, the person may be distracted, unfocused, and chaotic. It is a very vulnerable energy point and has to be protected. Massaging the navel can help release negative emotions, but massaging should only done around the navel rim and never inside the navel.

2. **Sexual Center:** In men this is called the Sperm Palace, which starts at the base of the penis. In women it's called the Ovarian Palace and is located above the pubic bone. To find the Ovarian Palace, place your thumbs on your navel and make the index fingers come together below. Where two index fingers meet is the location of the Ovarian Palace. The area where the pinkie fingers naturally touch is where ovaries are located. Sexual energy is the only energy that can be transformed into the life force and multiplied. When this energy is not used for procreation, it is easily lost through excessive sexual activity. In Taoist practice there are techniques that allow us to conserve this energy and use it for

healing and regeneration. When this center is open, the person is creative and playful. If this center is blocked, life's pleasures are drying out.

3. **Perineum, or the Gate of Life and Death:** Located between the anus and the sexual organ, the perineum is a very important point connected to the pelvic floor. If the pelvic floor is weak, this point is where the life force may leak out. If the pelvic floor is strong, a person can use the muscle of the pelvic floor to draw energy into the body. The perineum has a close connection to earth energy. When this point is open, the person feels grounded and secure. If it is blocked, the person feels insecure and unsure of herself.

4. **Sacrum:** In the Microcosmic Orbit there are two points connected to the sacrum, the tailbone and the sacrum itself. It's easier to just focus on the sacrum and let the energy flow from the perineum up the tailbone and up the sacrum. The sacrum is considered a pump that moves spinal fluid to the brain. Moving the base of the spine and using the mind to move energy up the spine helps keep the brain young and vibrant. The sacrum is connected to the earth force, the original force, so activating its energy by tapping or massaging this area can increase one's life force and vibrancy.

5. **Kidney center, or the Door of Life:** This center is located on the spine opposite the navel and corresponds to the lumbar vertebrae 2 and 3 (L2 and L3). This point is connected to our prenatal energy, which is the original force. When people live in stress and fear they deplete this energy, and this weakens the entire body. The kidney's energy can be replenished with Inner Smile Chi Kung, described in chapter 4, and with the Upward Draw of Sexual Energy, which is part of Taoist Healing Love practices described in the next chapter.

6. **Adrenal gland center:** The adrenal gland center is located on the spine at thoracic vertebra 11 (T11), opposite the solar plexus center. This center is controlled by the adrenal glands and is very

sensitive to stress. Its energy can be quickly drained by stimulants and drugs. When the adrenal center is open, life feels easy and free. When it is closed, life is difficult and blocked.

7. **Center opposite the heart:** This center is located on the spine, at thoracic 11 (T11), opposite the heart center. This center is closely connected to the heart and can contribute to creating the heart's radiance and shining. When this center is open, its energy protects the heart and the person experiences feelings of freedom, hope, and purpose. When it is blocked, the person will tend to feel melancholy, blocked, confused, and weighed down.

8. **Point opposite the throat:** This point is easy to find by locating the big protruding vertebra at the base of the neck, which is cervical vertebra 7 (C7). This point connects energy from the body to energy in the higher energy centers in the brain. If this point is blocked, energy may flow into the arms instead of going to the brain. When the C7 point is open, it is easier to connect with other people with compassion. If this point is blocked, people often feel inadequate and restricted in their expressions.

9. **Small brain point, or Jade Pillow:** This point is located above the last cervical vertebra at the base of the skull. It is connected to breathing, and when it is open it is believed that it helps us receive insights from the universe. This point is connected to the crown and third eye and stores yin energy. If this point is open but not connected to other points, too much energy can enter the brain, causing delusions and pressure. Opening the Microcosmic Orbit prevents this and ensures an even distribution of energy.

10. **Crown and Crystal Palace:** The crown point is located at the top of the head. To find this point, draw a line connecting the tips of the ears and going through the highest point of the head, and another line starting from the point between the two eyebrows all the way up to the base of the skull. This is an important energy point of connection to the forces of the universe.

Below the crown lies the Crystal Palace, which is where all the major brain glands are located, including the pineal gland, the pituitary gland, the thalamus, and the hypothalamus. When the Crystal Palace is activated, it illuminates the entire head, providing clarity, inner guidance, and insights. If the Crystal Palace is blocked, it can lead to delusions, confusion, and lack of direction.

11. **Mideyebrow point and Third Eye point:** The mideyebrow point is energetically connected to the pituitary gland, while the third eye point in the middle of the forehead is connected to the pineal gland. These two points can be used together as one center. The collective location of the important endocrine glands in the brain corresponds to the Taoist Crystal Palace in the middle of the brain. The Third Eye and the Mid-Eyebrow points enable connection to higher wisdom and universal light. When these points are activated, it's easier to get wisdom and insights. When they are closed, it's difficult to make decisions.

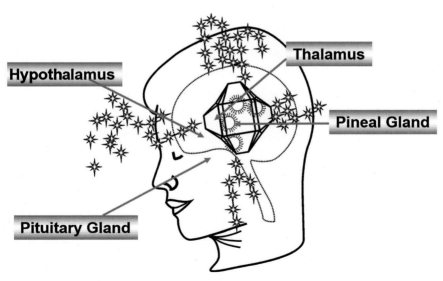

Figure 8.9. The crown point and the Crystal Palace, which includes the pineal gland, pituitary gland, thalamus, and hypothalamus.

12. **Heavenly Pool:** This is the point located on the roof of the mouth. When you place the tip of your tongue there, the two channels, yin and yang, become one orbit. There are three positions of the tongue: the wind position, located behind the front teeth; the fire position, which connects to the heart energy and is located further back on the palate; and the water position at the back. Usually, in the beginning it is easier to start with the Wind position. It can be activated by pressing the tip of the tongue to the roof of the mouth repeatedly.

13. **Throat point:** This point is located in the V-shaped space between the two collarbones. The throat point is connected to speech and communication. In Taoist philosophy, the tongue is a sense organ of the heart, and the throat point serves as an important energy bridge between the two. When this point is open, it is easier to express yourself with clarity and confidence. When it is closed, expression and communication become more difficult.

14. **Heart center:** The heart energy center on the Microcosmic Orbit is located on a direct line between the navel and the throat center, one inch above the tip of the sternum. The heart center can be opened with love, joy, and happiness. Massaging this area and practicing the heart sound also helps. For women, the heart center is very important because, according to Taoist teachings, a woman's heart center has to be open in order for her sexual energy to flow without blockages. For all sexes and genders, opening the heart center helps create radiance, beauty, and a connection to universal love.

15. **Solar plexus center:** The solar plexus center is located halfway between the heart center and the navel. It is connected to the spleen, pancreas, stomach, and liver. A strong solar plexus deters negative emotions and radiates a strong aura, like a little sun. This center can be strengthened by imagining sunshine radiating from this point. When it is open, the person feels daring and bold, and when it is closed, the person may be more fearful and unsure.

16. **Point under the knees:** This point can store additional spiritual energy.

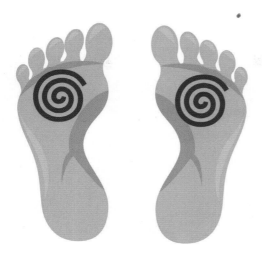

Figure 8.10.
Bubbling Springs point

17. **Bubbling Springs point:** This point is located on the soles of both feet, in the soft spot or depression on the sole. This point can draw in the earth force and is important for practicing grounding and stability.

18. **Big toe:** This point is on the lateral side of each big toe and it helps balance spiritual energy.

19. **Kneecap:** This point is in the middle of the upper portion of both knees. It helps refine earth energy as it goes up the legs.

The Microcosmic Orbit takes some time to open, but once it is open it runs by itself. All that's needed is to check the orbit from time to time to ensure that it is still running.

In addition to practicing the Microcosmic Orbit to balance and strengthen chi, the physical movements of Chi Kung work on the physical body to improve circulation, flexibility, and strength, as well as on the energy body by moving chi through the physical body. Physical Chi Kung practice also works on the mind, or information body, by honing our ability to guide our mind and build discipline and mental stamina. Physical Chi Kung practices such as those described in Master Chia's books *Healing Light of the Tao* and *Iron Shirt Chi Kung* are best done in the morning, but can be adjusted, depending on one's time.

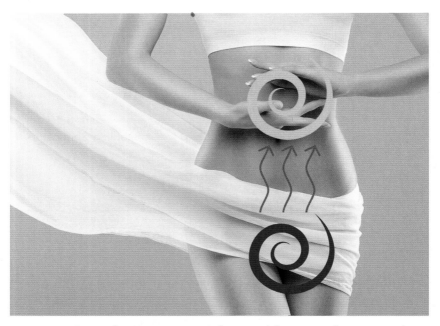

Figure 8.11. The Microcosmic Orbit can deliver sexual energy and unconditional love to all the organs and cells of the body.

Microcosmic Orbit Meditation

The Microcosmic Orbit starts and ends at the navel. It unites you as an integrated whole, with mind, body, and spirit flowing together, elevating your energy. Before you begin, review all nineteen points of the Microcosmic Orbit and locate them on your body. Walk yourself through all of them mentally, and then physically tap them if they are easy to access, and breathe into the points that are more difficult to reach. To move energy, use your smile, your eyes, and your mind to guide chi. The more you learn to focus inwardly and the more you learn to smile and relax, the more you will feel how real chi moves through your body, bringing light and life to all the organs and cells. First you learn to move your energy in the Small Moon Orbit (described below), then you expand it to a bigger Microcosmic Orbit, and finally, you can expand it even farther, in a Macrocosmic Orbit.

✺ Small Moon Orbit

1. Start by shaking your body to activate energy flow. Shake while standing up, relaxing your body and making all the joints loose and open.

2. Take a few deep abdominal breaths, inhaling while pushing the abdomen out and exhaling while pulling the navel toward the spine.

3. Rock your spine and imagine you have a dragon tail grounding you into the earth. Visualize deep roots growing from the soles of your feet into the earth.

4. Sit straight on the edge of a chair. Take a few deep breaths and relax. Turn your mind inward. Start by smiling into your heart with love, joy, and happiness.

5. Bring your attention to your navel and smile into it. Become aware of your abdominal fire. Feel your navel getting warm and flowing. Imagine a ball of energy rotating behind your navel.

6. Exhale the ball of energy to your pubic bone, guiding it with your mind's eyes and your smile. Breathe into your pubic bone and smile into it. You can use your hands to guide energy down from your navel.

7. Exhale the energy down to your perineum. Smile into your perineum. Inhale, keeping the energy in your perineum, then pull your perineum up and exhale, relaxing your body. Some people find it helpful to sit on a tennis ball to bring more awareness to this point.

8. Gently tap your tailbone. Smile into your tailbone. Inhale and use your mind and intention to pull energy up your tailbone. Keep your chest relaxed. It's very important to be very gentle with yourself and stay within your comfort zone.

9. Gently tap your sacrum. Smile into your sacrum. Inhale into your tailbone and pull energy up your sacrum, then exhale and relax, smiling into your sacrum.

10. Gently tap your Door of Life (the point on your spine across from your navel). Smile into your Door of Life. Inhale into your sacrum and pull energy up to your Door of Life. Exhale, relax, smile, and rock your spine. Then connect your Door of Life with your navel and move the energy into your navel, completing a small orbit. Use

both hands to guide the energy down the midline again, to the pubic bone and to the perineum, and then up the sacrum again.

◉ Microcosmic Orbit

1. Begin at your navel and move your energy down to your perineum and up to your Door of Life. Then smile into your adrenal gland center (the point on your spine across from your solar plexus) and imagine pulling the energy up your spine to your adrenal gland center. Exhale, relax, and smile.

2. Smile into the area on your spine across from your heart center. This is the Wing Point. Inhale and pull the energy up to this point. Exhale, smile, and relax.

3. Gently tap the point opposite the throat, on the protruding neck vertebrae (C7). Smile into your C7. Inhale and pull energy up to this point. Exhale, smile, and relax.

4. Gently tap the base of your skull and smile into your Jade Pillow. Pull energy up into the Jade Pillow.

5. Smile into your crown and put your tongue on the roof of your mouth. There are three locations on the roof of your mouth—front (behind the teeth), middle, and back. Explore which one allows for a more noticeable energy flow. Later you may practice alternating all of them. Guide chi up to your crown.

6. Smile down into your third eye and into your physical eyes. Imagine your eyes becoming cooler and more relaxed. Then smile and let chi flow down through your sinuses to the roof of your mouth, to your tongue, throat, heart center, and solar plexus, and finally to your navel. Keep the energy moving through this orbit, directing it with your attention and focus. Remember to smile and relax.

7. When you're done, collect chi in your navel by massaging your belly around the outside of your navel (not in the naval) twenty-four times counterclockwise, expanding the spiral. Then massage in the opposite direction, thirty-six times, concentrating energy in the navel. Imagine there is a small cauldron in your navel where you collect energy.

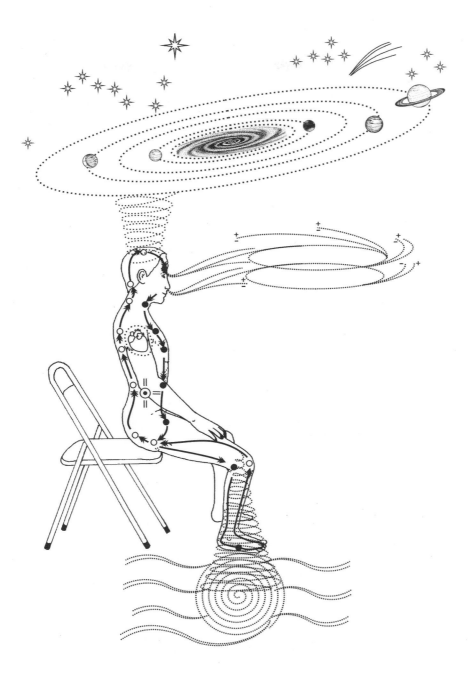

Figure 8.12.
The Microcosmic Orbit.

8. When you become more familiar with moving the orbit through your body, you can expand it from your perineum to the soles of your feet, and then up your legs and into your perineum again. The orbit flows in a figure eight pattern, so when you reach the perineum, moving from the navel, you continue from the perineum down the back of your thighs to the points under your knees and down to the Bubbling Springs, and then to your big toe point and up the front of your legs to your kneecap point and then back to your perineum, to continue up your tailbone and up your spine.

Eventually all you will need to do is to think about your orbit and send energy flowing, and it will flow like a river, nourishing your whole body. Remember, your skin drinks from the same reservoir of energy as all your other organs. Take good care of your energy, and your energy will take good care of your skin, your body, and your beauty. The Microcosmic Orbit eventually becomes the Macrocosmic Orbit, or Cosmic Orbit,[9] where

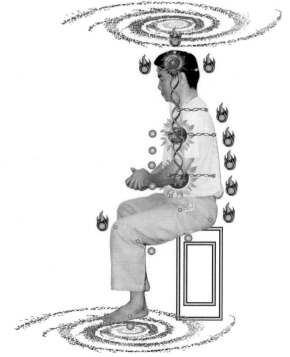

Figure 8.13.
The Macrocosmic Orbit.

you let the figure eight pattern continue to include the sun, the moon, and the planets, as well as the earth. This creates an expansive, radiant feeling and refines your energy. The more you practice the orbit, the more your skin will begin to glow and start looking younger and more relaxed. The Microcosmic Orbit is also called the Healing Light meditation because you are letting the light, or chi, move through your body, energizing and clearing negative energy and blockages.

Once you've become familiar with the route of the Microcosmic Orbit, you can check to see if it runs well by simply guiding your consciousness from your navel to your perineum on an exhalation, then from your perineum to your crown on an inhalation, and then from your crown down the midline to your navel on an exhalation. Once the Microcosmic Orbit is open and running, there is no need to think about the specific points. If certain points seem to be blocked and feel like the flow is not even, you will need to tap the points (where you can reach them), smile, and breathe into them. This way if you catch any blockages early enough you can easily open them before they grow bigger and create stagnation. The Microcosmic Orbit is the main energy highway, and all the other energy channels are connected to it. It takes very little effort to check it, and doing so can bring great benefits.

The Microcosmic Orbit helps us avoid a congestion of negative emotions, so we're less likely to have uncontrolled outbursts of anger or unexpected tears. When the skin is well-nourished by chi and emotional energy doesn't build up, we have a more relaxed, youthful, pleasant, and composed expression. In addition, the Microcosmic Orbit is the essential path for moving sexual energy to the brain and to the organs. Since sexual energy is the most powerful energy, and when combined with unconditional love it has exceptional healing powers, it is essential to take care of the Microcosmic Orbit to ensure that the body's most powerful beauty elixir is delivered and distributed to every cell in the body.

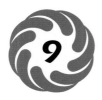

Sexual Energy Cultivation for Beauty

The radiant glow and vibrancy of young skin is its most attractive quality. Young skin heals quickly, can tolerate more stress and neglect compared to aged skin without losing its beauty, and has a special, unmistakably fresh and vital energy. Taoists discovered that beauty and vitality, not only of the skin but of the entire body, can be increased through the healing and invigorating power of sexual energy. According to the Tao, sexual energy is the most powerful creative and healing force there is, and when we learn to protect and conserve it, we can use it for healing and revitalization of the skin and the entire body. Sexual energy is not the same as sexual desire, sexual pleasure, or arousal. Sexual energy is the essential energy that Taoists call *Ching* (or *Jing*), which every human being receives at the moment of conception, and which is stored and produced in the sexual organs.

In a male body, Ching is used to generate sperm and infuse it with enough life force to conceive a fetus, and in a female body it is used for ovulation, menstruation, the development of an ovum, the growth of a fetus in the womb, and for breastfeeding a newborn. This energy is also used for creative endeavors and expressions. Ching can be transformed into chi, which can be used to supply energy to the organs and tissues; it can be also refined and transformed into spiritual energy, which Taoists call *Chen*.

Qualities of Feminine Sexual Energy

- It is connected to the water element and the color blue.
- It is nurturing and life-giving.
- It is yin in its passive state and yang during arousal.
- It is connected to playfulness and creativity.
- It is resilient.
- It is mainly generated in the ovaries, but also in the breasts, yoni (i.e., vagina), and uterus.
- It is heavy and dense, so it tends to accumulate in the lower parts of the body.
- It is essential for giving more power to the higher energy centers and supporting the brain.
- Orgasmic energy combined with unconditional love makes the most powerful healing elixir.

Qualities of Male Sexual Energy

- When stored, it is connected to the wood element when at rest and to fire when aroused. According to Tao Masters, male sexual energy is quick to arouse just as wood is quick to catch fire.
- Sexual energy activates first, which activates the flow of the heart energy.
- It is the source of creativity and vitality, just like female sexual energy.
- It is stored in testicles and is lost with semen during ejaculation. Therefore Taoist practices for men are aimed at preserving the semen and returning sexual energy to the organs.

It is important to notice that both biological males and biological females have male and female sexual energy. To aid in healing the body and rejuvenating the skin, men, just like women, are advised to cultivate their female sexual energy, which has the nourishing qualities of the water element. This means relaxation, softness, and gentleness in flow. In the highest Taoist practices, students learn to embrace and combine their male and female essences.[1]

THE ROLE OF FEMALE SEX HORMONES IN THE SKIN

Taoist masters did not know modern biology, however they were correct when they made the connection between a woman's vitality and her sexual energy. Today Western science knows that estrogen is responsible for the development of the female sexual organs as well as the external female characteristics of the body and the sexual drive; estrogen also has a profound and beneficial effect on a woman's skin. As a general principle, an imbalance or excess—whether of estrogen or anything else for that matter—has negative consequences for one's health and vitality, so both an excess or a deficiency of estrogen can have negative consequences for the skin's beauty, health, and radiance.

Importantly, both women and men have estrogen, the female sex hormone (yin), as well as androgen, the male sexual hormone (yang).

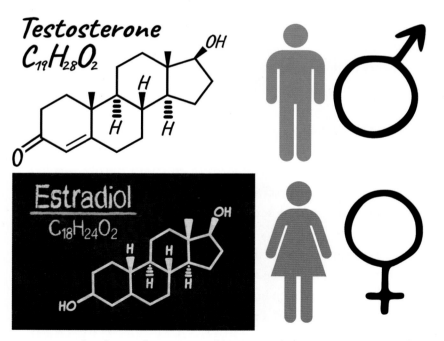

Figure 9.1. The chemical structures of beta-estradiol (i.e., estrogen, the female sex hormone) and testosterone (the male sex hormone)

There are three main forms of estrogen: estrone, estradiol, and estriol, while the main androgen is testosterone. Women typically have low levels of testosterone, usually anywhere from 9 to 55 ng/dL (nanograms per deciliter), while men have from 300 to 1,000 ng/dL of testosterone. The reason why women's bodies have much less testosterone is because in female tissues the male hormone is converted into estradiol by an enzyme called *aromatase.*

Most people know that sex hormones are produced in the sexual organs—the testicles in men and the ovaries in women. But it was not until 1974 that researchers discovered that estrogen is also produced in adipose (fat) tissue.[2] Since then it's been confirmed that estrogen is also produced in the skin, brain, liver, bones, and the adrenal glands.[3]

In menopause, when estrogen production starts declining, the impact on a woman's body will greatly depend on how well these other sites of estrogen production work. If the skin can make enough estrogen and distribute it to its cells, the woman will have smoother, brighter, more resilient skin.

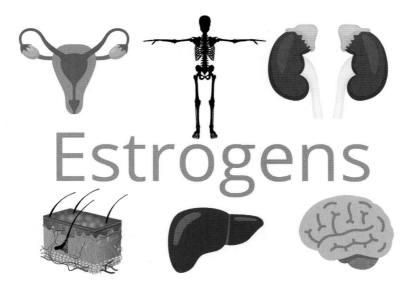

Figure 9.2. Estrogen is produced in the ovaries, bones, adrenal glands, skin, liver, brain, and fatty tissue.

The skin not only makes its own sex hormones, it is also very responsive to them. Female and male sex hormones (yin and yang) have opposite effects on the skin. The female sexual hormone, estrogen, balances skin oil production, while the male sexual hormone, androgen, increases skin oiliness and aggravates acne in women. Estrogen makes sure the skin is not too oily and not too dry. The decrease in female sexual hormones in menopause can result in increased overall dryness of the skin and an increase of oil production locally. Female sexual hormones in both sexes balance the synthesis of collagen and glycosaminoglycans, and ensure the regeneration of skin cells. This is why young women who have not yet experienced the hormonal imbalance brought on by menopause tend to have smooth, glowing skin with small pores and an elastic, resilient texture. On the other hand, an active form of testosterone called *dihydrotestosterone,* or DHT, in the skin is responsible for acne, excessive oiliness, and hair loss. Skin changes in menopause result from both a deficiency of estrogen and an increase of testosterone. The less testosterone is converted to estrogen in the ovaries, the more it is present in the skin and the rest of the body. Also, estrogen counteracts the effects of testosterone (i.e., yin and yang balance), so when estrogen starts declining, testosterone is free to influence the skin, causing problems like clogged pores and facial hair.

The Effects of Estrogen Deficiency on the Skin

- Accelerates aging, increases sagging
- More facial hair due to increased testosterone
- Fragmented collagen, fewer glycosaminoglycans
- Slower wound healing
- Dullness and dryness
- Thinner and more fragile skin
- Enlarged and clogged pores

The Effects of Estrogen Excess in the Skin (such as during pregnancy)

- Increased pigmentation
- Stretch marks
- Possible increase of hormone-related cancers such as breast cancer

Many women notice that once they turn fifty and start approaching menopause, their skin starts aging much faster. Their eyes may become hollow and crow's feet may become deeper. Aging is a physiological process, with real physiological changes that need to be taken into account. Women cannot just wish menopause away, they have to go through it. So it is important to know how to support the mind, body, and spirit during this time.

Many do not realize that estrogen is not just a sex hormone. It supports the synthesis of collagen in the skin and influences metabolism and therefore affects energy level and body weight, brain health, and bone density. A decrease of estrogen in menopause results in many unpleasant symptoms such as vaginal dryness, hot flashes, skin irritations, forgetfulness, emotional instability, depression, and increased risk of fractures. Many women start losing bladder control when they sneeze, cough, or laugh, due to the weakening of the pelvic diaphragm, which has muscle and connective tissue that contains collagen and elastin. When collagen synthesis declines, the pelvic floor starts weakening. Women may experience thinning of the hair or noticeable hair loss during menopause. Some women adjust to these changes more easily, but others may feel unattractive, old, undesirable, and unworthy. These emotions affect the skin's radiance, vitality, and beauty more than the effects of aging.

Hormone Replacement Therapy (HRT) has been shown to improve collagen density and content, increase skin vitality and thickness, and generally make the skin look younger and more radiant. However many women do not want to take artificial hormones, which have known adverse effects on the body. It is important to understand that natural estrogen, produced in the body, and artificial estrogen, which is used in HRT, are not the same. Natural estrogen is highly beneficial and has so many supportive and protective functions that some poetically call it a protective umbrella that nature holds over female bodies. A popular option is phytoestrogens, which are bioactive chemicals naturally found in plants such as red clover, soybeans, yam, red grapes, and others. Phytoestrogens work by binding to the same receptors that are used for estrogen. A receptor is a protein in a cell's membrane that works as a switch to trigger a biochemical response. Phytoestrogens work as a very weak form of natural estrogen, so there is little to no risk of any side effects. They can also support the skin through their antioxidant and anti-inflammatory actions.[4]

There are three main classes of phytoestrogens: isoflavones, lignans, and coumestans, all of which have been confirmed to have positive effects on aging skin as well as in alleviating some common symptoms of menopause.

Classes of Phytoestrogens

- Isoflavones such as daidzein and genistein are natural compounds found in soybeans and other legumes.
- Lignans such as enterodiol and enterolactone are found in legumes, berries, seeds (particularly flaxseed), grains, nuts, and fruits.
- Coumestans such as coumestrol are found in red clover, alfalfa, and spinach.

ESTROGEN AND MENTAL HEALTH

"Why I am so exhausted all the time? I used to have so much energy." This is a very common complaint heard from women over fifty. Some women try to push through the situation, generating a lot of worry and anxiety in the process. What they don't realize is that this drop in energy level and stress resilience is connected to hormonal changes. Female sex hormones make us more resilient, increasing our ability to manage stress and pain. This helps a woman get through pregnancy, labor, and breastfeeding, as well as all the challenges of raising a child. Once estrogen starts declining with age, the body's stress resilience goes down too. If a woman continues to expend energy the way she used to, burning through her reserves, it can have devastating effects on her skin. Many professional women who have relied on their ability to push through stress and fatigue may start feeling exhausted when they never have before. And exhaustion is never good for the skin.

Estrogen has a protective effect against age-related cognitive decline and neurodegeneration. The brain fog and forgetfulness that many women over fifty may start experiencing is believed to be caused by a decline of estrogen. Stress adds to it. Today it is universally accepted that mental fog and forgetfulness are among the many symptoms of menopause. This doesn't have to be, though. In the past, elderly medicine women, witches, and shamans were revered for their wisdom and mental powers. The Tao believes that any woman who wants to be vital, beautiful, and mentally clear must to learn to cultivate her sexual energy and take care of chi flow in her reproductive organs.

SEXUAL ENERGY CULTIVATION PRINCIPLES

Taoist sexual energy cultivation practices are based on the premise that both men and women can be renewed and invigorated by cultivating their sexual energy, since it is the very energy that creates life. A healthy man can ejaculate from 200 to 500 hundred million sperm in one go, but it only takes one sperm to fertilize an egg. A million-to-one chance is nothing compared to winning the incredible cosmic lottery of conception! Taoists hold that when a sperm makes its way to an egg and they merge, they vibrate love and orgasmic energy, which attracts a massive charge of cosmic energy, the primordial creative force. According to Taoist teachings, when we are conceived we receive 100 percent of this primordial life force.

At the moment of conception, the primordial life force is divided into three parts: 50 percent goes to the overall life force; 25 percent goes to fuel sexual energy, to ensure that you can procreate and pass on your genetic material; and 25 percent is reserved for emergencies and stored in the kidneys, to use only when the body is hurt, unwell, or under attack. Each of us is born with a certain amount of genetically determined life force, or chi, to spend on everyday activities, work, fun, and various physiological functions. We can replenish chi by converting food into energy; however even digesting food to generate energy requires energy. So when the life force is depleted, it becomes more difficult to generate energy.

According to the Tao, some people are born with abundant energy, while others may be given a more limited supply. Like winning the cosmic lottery, some people get a big win and can spend lavishly all their life, while others have a limited win and can therefore risk spending it too quickly. The key is to use it wisely. Just because someone is gifted

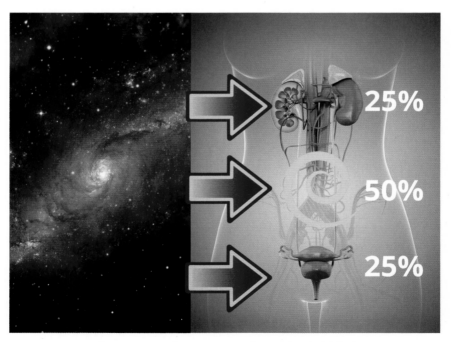

Figure 9.3. At the moment of conception, the primordial life force is divided to three parts: 50 percent goes to the life force, 25 percent to sexual energy, and 25 percent is reserved for emergencies, where it is stored in the kidneys.

with abundant energy does not mean it is wise to burn through their fortune too quickly. According to the Tao, the kidneys store our gold reserve of energy. This energy is released if we are injured, ill, stressed, or are being chased by a big lion. Stressful and frightening events can trigger a release of adrenaline from the adrenal glands, located on top of the kidneys. Adrenaline helps mobilize energy and increases our ability to fight or flee—a healthy reaction. But under chronic stress many women burn up their energy reserves in the kidneys, leaving themselves unprotected in case of an injury or illness. Perhaps some people think that being constantly stressed helps them deal with problems in some way, but problems never end, and if they never return the energy they borrow from the kidneys, they will drain their reserves.

Sexual energy can also be transformed into negative energy. When too much negative energy is stored in the sexual organs, the flow of sexual energy becomes blocked and stagnates, with excessive energy

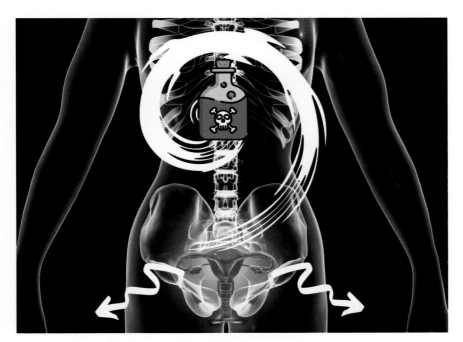

Figure 9.4. Sexual energy can be transformed into negative emotional energy or lost.

accumulating in the organs and depletion of sexual energy occurring in the rest of the body. Sexual energy can also be lost through sex, excessive sexual desire, and stimulation of the senses. When negative energy is transformed back into life force and flow is restored, the person can return to balance.

The more a person learns to relax and bring balance into their life, the more energy they will have in reserve to deal with life's inevitable challenges. A reserve of life force is even more crucial as we age because our body needs more energy to repair and regenerate. Fully 25 percent of our total life force energy is stored in the sexual organs to be used for reproduction. It takes a lot of life force to grow a human being! Since procreation is so important, nature made sure people have enough energy to make it possible to have a baby every year. Some of this energy is lost every month through menstruation, while some of it is used to breastfeed a baby (or a few babies). Nowadays most women limit themselves to one to three children, and even if they have five or six kids it's still way less than what nature has prepared the female body for.

This means that even in menopause a female body still has plenty of sexual energy in reserve. Taoists say that sexual energy is the only energy that can be transformed back into the life force. Instead of wasting and exhausting one's sexual energy, we can learn to use it to have more uplifting, vibrant, and vital energy overall. When we're young we're energy millionaires and can spend lavishly, never concerning ourselves with wasting our life force or our sexual energy. We have plenty. When we get older and our life force starts getting lower, many people, especially highly ambitious women who want to continue being high producers, start using stress and worry to trick their body into releasing some of their emergency energy. It may feel good to feel this rush of adrenaline, however this is the very energy the body needs to hold in reserve to fight illness and deal with aging. Many women don't realize that the adrenal glands, which release adrenaline, also produce testosterone, which is responsible for many unpleasant effects, such as excessive facial hair and acne.

A woman's sexual organs, like every other organ in her body, need the energy provided by plenty of fresh, oxygenated blood flowing through every cell and through the muscles and fascia. To rejuvenate and reinvigorate, women need regular physical movement to activate chi flow and bring strength and power to the physical structures. The sexual organs are affected by emotional energy, which can be either life-giving or draining, so in addition to a regular physical exercise routine it is important to do regular energy clearing to ensure that the source of sexual energy is pure, clean, and nourishing. Shame, guilt, and grief, three destructive emotions that plague many women over fifty, can block sexual energy.

There is not much that modern Western medicine can offer to a woman to support her sexual energy. Western medicine is expensive, intrusive, and often quite impersonal. Of course it is important to note that there are cases when a conventional medical treatment may be necessary and life-saving. At the same time it is also important to understand

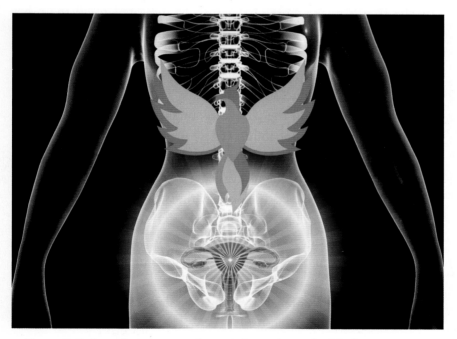

Figure 9.5. Sexual energy can be transformed into the life force to create radiance and vitality.

that when a woman is going through the challenges of aging and meno-pause, she needs the care and support of good nutrition, mental balance, and physical exercise. Considering the fact that estrogen is produced in the skin and fatty tissues, a woman may want to consider keeping a little extra body fat to support her estrogen production, which, compared to a thinner body, will result in stronger bones, healthier skin, less brain fog and fatigue, and overall a more sustainable energy level.[5]

Physical exercise that builds strong muscles should be done in mod-eration as a woman ages; is much more important to support energy flow and circulation through the soft tissues and ensure that the body is connected into an integrated system, through which estrogen and energy flows freely. All the practices discussed in the previous chapters are very useful in supporting the skin in menopause. The Inner Smile, described in chapter 4, and the Six Healing Sounds, found in chapter 7, help release negative energy and replenish the body with radiant and vibrant energy. Stem Cell Chi Kung, described in chapter 6, helps acti-vate the skin to make more estrogen to be delivered to all the other organs and tissues. And the Microcosmic Orbit, described in chapter 8, connects all the organs, including the sexual organs, the skin, and the brain, in one flow of enriching chi.

This chapter introduces a unique set of Taoist vitality practices for women and men that in the past were taught only to students of the Tao and to Emperor's concubines. These practices include meditation, mindful movements of Chi Kung, and, for women, if they wish, the use of a drilled egg carved from jade, called a *jade egg* or *yoni egg*. If you're new to these kinds of practices you may find some of them fall outside of your comfort zone. That's okay. Try the exercises that feel right for you and skip the others. While doing all of the practices will have the greatest benefit, even doing just one will make a difference.

All the practices presented in this chapter should be performed with full awareness and attention to the body. The authors are not medical professionals. Please consult your doctor if you have any medical issues of concern before undertaking these practices.

SEXUAL ENERGY CULTIVATION
PRACTICES FOR WOMEN

The sexual organs are capable of generating powerful energy. As long as they are strong and healthy, they can do it in perimenopause or even in postmenopause. When women reconnect with their feminine force, they reconnect to their intrinsic magic, power, and confidence. They start looking younger, more radiant, and more vital.

There are a number of Taoist practices that cultivate and direct feminine energy. It is very important to be mindful and pay close attention to body sensations while undertaking any of the following practices. As well, it is very important to be relaxed and smile into your body while doing these practices. The more you relax, the easier it is for energy to flow.

 ## Pelvic Floor Training

For more information, see *Healing Love through the Tao: Cultivating Female Sexual Energy* by Mantak Chia and Maneewan Chi.

1. Stand in the Chi Kung posture (as if you are about to sit, but do not sit) with your feet shoulder-width apart. Keep your spine straight and your lower abdomen open, with your tailbone slightly tucked in. Relax and feel your feet growing roots to ground you into the earth.
2. Slightly shake your body in smooth, relaxed movements of your limbs and spine.
3. Gently rotate your head to release your neck. Position your head on your neck as if there was a silk thread suspending your head such that there is absolutely no effort holding your head erect.
4. Smile into your body and wiggle your toes. Connect your toes to the ground.
5. Imagine your dragon tail growing into the ground. Feel grounded in your body.
6. Bring your attention to your anus. Remember a time when you felt the urgent need to go to the toilet to do a "number 2" but had to

hold it? Inhale, and just as if you needed to hold it, squeeze the circular muscle around your anus. Hold your breath for a moment, then relax, release, and smile into your anus. This is an important part of your body. According to the Tao, when the anus muscles get loose, we start losing energy. Repeat this movement nine times and keep smiling into this area.

7. Your anus has another muscle that lifts the anus. Inhale, pull your anus up, and hold your breath for a moment, then relax, release, and smile. Do this nine times.

8. Bring your attention to the left and then to the right side of your anus. Think of all the left-side organs sitting on your left anus. Pull the left side up and imagine it lifting the left-side organs up. Do the same with your right-side of your anus and the right-side organs. Do this nine times on each side.

9. Inhale and pull your perineum up. This is the space between your anus and your sexual organs. You can touch this area to increase your awareness. Exhale and relax. Repeat nine times.

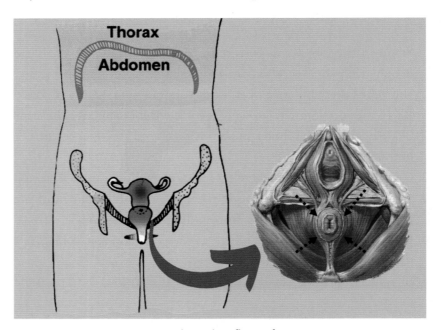

Figure 9.6. The pelvic floor of a woman.

Lotus Meditation, or Heart-to-Kidneys Breathing

Sexual energy is connected to the kidneys and to the element of water. This is a great calming and balancing practice for the entire body. The heart is often overheated with worry and anxiousness, while the kidneys are often cold because of too much fear and similar blockages. This affects sexual energy, which can become cold and stagnant. This meditation restores flow and infuses the skin with a beautiful glow.

1. Sit on the edge of a chair. Put your feet on the floor and feel connected to the earth. Take a few deep, relaxing breaths. Smile into your body.
2. Imagine your heart as a beautiful lotus flower absorbing the energy of the sun. Feel nice and warm in your heart. Smile into your heart.
3. Imagine your kidneys as the bulbous roots of the lotus flower floating in cool, clear water. Smile into your kidneys.

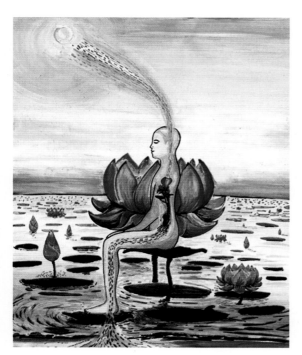

Figure 9.7.
The Lotus Meditation.

4. Imagine your feet are the roots of the lotus flower growing deep into the earth.

5. Smile into your heart and inhale. Exhale with the heart sound *haw-www* down into your kidneys. Feel warm heart energy flowing into your kidneys, warming them up.

6. Inhale from your kidneys and exhale all the way down to the earth through your "roots."

7. Inhale from your feet up and exhale into your kidneys.

8. Inhale from your kidneys and exhale with the kidneys the sound *chooooo,* all the way into the heart. Feel cool, watery energy flowing into the heart, cooling it down.

9. Keep breathing in this pattern at least nine times, feeling your heart and kidneys balancing their energy.

Ovarian Breathing Practice

This practice transforms negative energy stored in the ovaries back into healthy, free-flowing life force. It energizes and activates the ovaries, preventing energy blocks and stagnation.

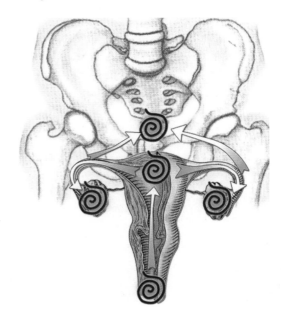

Figure 9.8.
Ovarian breathing.

1. Place your two thumbs on your navel and extend your two index fingers down toward your pubic bone. The place where your pinkie fingers meet is approximately where your ovaries are located.
2. Imagine your ovaries as two flowers that can open and close.
3. Imagine the mouth of your uterus (if you still have it, and if you don't, imagine connecting to the energy space of the uterus) as another flower that can open and close.
4. Keep your focus on this image and inhale, visualizing that you are inhaling into your ovaries. See your ovaries opening and taking the life force in.
5. Exhale, visualizing that you are exhaling from your ovaries. See your ovaries closing and releasing any dark and cloudy energy.

USING A YONI EGG TO CULTIVATE CHI

Because of its egg shape, the yoni egg is uniquely suited to help move energy in the vagina, or yoni, a woman's sacred space. This practice brings more awareness and energy to one's feminine energy and physical organs. The benefits include:

- **Better circulation and flow through mindfulness:** The yoni egg practice is done with mindfulness and inner focus, which supports the flow of chi and improves circulation.
- **Hydration of connective tissues:** The repeated squeezing and releasing action of the practice trains the muscles, releases tension, hydrates the tissues, and activates lymphatic flow. There is no substitute for this valuable practice.
- **Better focus:** The physical presence of an egg in the yoni helps bring awareness and focus into this area. It makes it easy to visualize what you cannot see while it helps the mind send healing energy to the reproductive system.
- **Lymphatic massage and detox:** The yoni egg creates a gentle massaging action that improves circulation and blood flow, helping to remove toxins and negative energy.

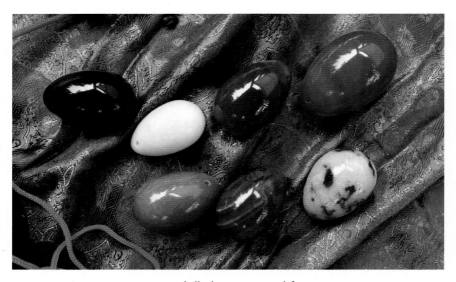

Figure 9.9. Yoni eggs are drilled eggs carved from various gemstones.

- **Energy clearing:** The yoni egg is made of a natural gemstone, jade, which is an earth element, therefore it absorbs negative energy from the sexual organs. The egg is easy to clean by washing it thoroughly and placing it under the moonlight.
- **Facilitates overall healing:** Sexual energy cultivation practices give women control over their most powerful force, enabling them to direct it to other areas that may need healing.
- **Helps the brain stay vibrant:** The yoni egg practice involves moving sexual energy up the spine to replenish the highest energy center, which adds vibrant life force to the brain.

You can purchase yoni eggs from the Tao Garden in Thailand to ensure their good quality, or find a reputable seller. The egg should be carved from natural stone such as jade and definitely should not be painted. These eggs come in small, medium, and large sizes. You might want to start with a medium-size egg to see how it feels. A stone can be any stone, but many women like to pick a stone that resonates with their energy. Refer to books about gemstones to choose your egg, or just purchase whatever stone appeals to you.

Yoni Egg Practice

Note: We highly recommend you work with a certified Universal Healing Tao Healing Love instructor to guide you through the following practice. But if you do it on your own, please read the instructions carefully and listen to your body. There should be no pain or discomfort involved. Do not do this practice if you have any medical condition such as an infection or inflammation.

1. Before using your egg, wash it thoroughly with soap and very hot water. Some advise boiling some water, turning the heat off, and then placing the egg in the water for a a period of time to sterilize it. As well, make sure you wash your egg after using it. Store it in a clean, dry place. You might consider putting it in the sunlight or moonlight once in a while to clear its energy and recharge it.

2. If your stone comes with a string, toss the string because you are going to use dental floss (original, not mint) instead, and discard the string after each use. Simply take a length of floss approximately the length your elbow to the end of your fingers. Fold the floss in two and thread the folded end through the hole in the egg. Now you have a loop on one end and two loose ends on the other end of the hole. Now thread the loose ends through the loop and let it tighten. The egg is now secure, with enough length to hold the egg.

3. Warm your egg in your hands before inserting it. Put it on your heart area and breathe love into it.

4. You can use a lubricant in your yoni or on the egg (whichever is easier for you) before inserting the egg into your yoni. It should go in easily, without any effort. Gently place its blunt end at the entrance of your yoni and guide it in while lying on your back.

5. When the egg is in, gently pull the attached string to alert your body that there is something that needs attention. At this stage, pull the string very gently, keeping the egg inside.

6. Relax and smile into your yoni. Become aware of the egg and see it with your mind's eye. Breathe into your yoni.

7. Gently squeeze and pull your anus and perineum up as you inhale. Imagine your vagina gently squeezing the egg. Exhale and relax. If your yoni is already strong enough, the egg will start moving up because of its shape. If the egg doesn't move, just keep practicing every day for a few minutes until you feel it moving. Be patient.

8. When the egg starts moving you'll know it, because the loose end of the floss (the string) will start moving in your fingers. At this stage you are ready for the next step. Gently pull the string as you exhale a long cleansing breath and let the egg move down almost to the entrance of your yoni. Then move it up again. Repeat 9 times.

9. When you are ready to complete this practice, gently pull the egg all the way out. Smile into your yoni and think love, joy, happiness, and gratitude. Wash the egg and store it in a clean, dry place.

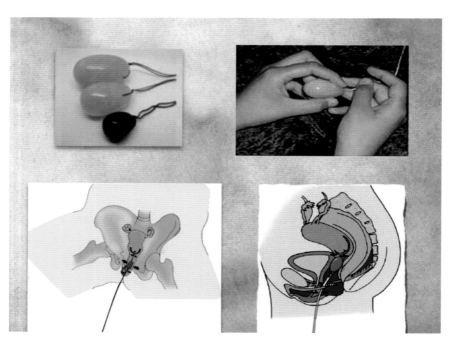

Figure 9.10. The yoni egg practice.

Breast Massage

As part of the female reproductive system, the breasts can generate sexual energy. Activating the flow of chi in the breast area restores their connection to the pelvic sexual organs and ensures that the whole body has a good, strong flow of energy. This helps prevent your breasts from sagging and keeps the skin in the décolleté area stronger, more vibrant, and more resilient.

The breasts are often restricted by garments and a slouched posture. Breasts have a complex lymphatic and circulatory system designed by nature to ensure milk production. Once there is no need to make milk, breast circulation may become clogged and stagnant. Breast massage helps transform sexual energy stored in the breasts into life force energy.

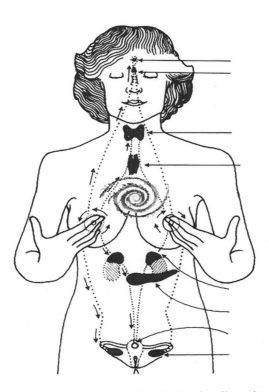

Figure 9.11. Breast massage can replenish the décolleté skin of the chest, neck, shoulders, and back, and also firm the breasts.

1. Hold your palms under your breasts. Start gently moving your palms in an inward circular motion, massaging the breasts with slight pressure. You can add massage oil for enjoyment and better movement. Do nine circles around each breast.

2. After you've completed nine inward circles, reverse direction and massage in outward circles.

3. Massage your nipples. This activates contractions in the uterus (if you have one, and if you don't, visualize the energy space of the uterus) and helps restore energy flow. Remember to smile, keeping your body relaxed, and be very gentle.

4. Using gentle spiraling movements of your palms, massage down along the line that connects your breasts and your pubic bone. Taoists believe that this line still retains energy connections from our mammalian past, when the female body had additional milk glands on the abdomen.

5. Finish by holding your breasts and gently shaking them to activate chi flow.

Female Upward Draw of Sexual Energy

This practice builds on the previous practices and connects sexual energy flow to the higher energy centers. In this practice you will generate sexual energy in your perineum, build it up, and then direct it into the Microcosmic Orbit. Review the Microcosmic Orbit in the previous chapter before starting this practice. The Upward Draw is used in Taoist Healing Love practices,* which preserve and redirect orgasmic energy to be used for healing and spiritual growth. Instead of allowing orgasm to pour out

---

*Taoist Healing Love practices are further explored in Master Chia's *Healing Love through the Tao: Cultivating Female Sexual Energy.* You are also encouraged to find a certified Universal Healing Tao instructor or take classes with Master Chia. The more you learn about how to draw your sexual energy upward to turn it into a river of chi, the more you will increase the shining glow and healthful radiance of your skin.

of the body, it is directed up the spine and into the Microcosmic Orbit. Then it can be safely stored in the navel cauldron for future use by massaging the abdomen in a spiral motion—first from the navel outwardly and then from the outer edge of the abdomen spiraling inwardly gathering the energy in the navel.

1. You can do this practice sitting, standing, or lying down.
2. Bring your attention to your perineum and smile into it. Relax, inhale, and pull your perineum up. Hold for a few seconds. Exhale and release.
3. Repeat step 2 at least nine times. Feel your perineum becoming warm and more alive.
4. Rest and keep your focus on your perineum. Feel it becoming warmer.
5. Repeat step 2 at least nine more times. You can do it for a total of eighteen or thirty-six times.
6. Rest, focus with your physical and inner eyes, and smile into your perineum. Feel your perineum becoming warmer.
7. Spiral your physical eyes, your inner eyes, and your mind in your perineum, gathering the energy there into a chi ball.
8. Inhale up the spine, rolling your eyes up, pulling energy up your tailbone. Exhale and feel the ball of energy spinning in your sacrum.
9. Inhale the ball of energy and roll your eyes up to the Door of Life. Exhale and feel the ball of energy spinning in your Door of Life.
10. Inhale the ball of energy and roll your eyes up to your adrenal gland center. Exhale and feel the ball of energy spinning in your adrenal gland center.
11. Inhale the ball of energy and roll your eyes up to the point opposite your heart. Exhale and feel the ball of energy spinning in this point.
12. Inhale the ball of energy and roll your eyes up to the cervical vertebra at the base of your neck, C7. Exhale and feel the ball of energy spinning in C7.
13. Inhale the ball of energy and roll your eyes up to the small brain point at the base of your neck, the Jade Pillow. Tap the back of the skull and exhale and feel the ball of energy spinning in this point.

14. Inhale the ball of energy and roll your eyes up to your crown. Exhale and spiral the ball of chi under your crown with your eyes.

15. Exhale and guide the energy down through your third eye, sinuses, throat center, heart center, and solar plexus, into your navel. Spiral your eyes like a vortex and spin the ball of chi in your navel.

16. Finish this practice by gathering chi in your navel and massaging outward from your navel in an expanding spiral thirty-six times, and then reverse the direction and spiral inward twenty-four times, condensing the spiral down into your navel.

17. Rest and feel your body replenished and rejuvenated.

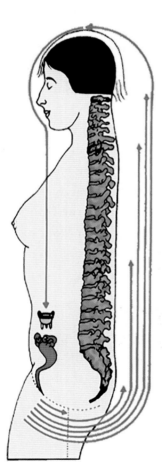

Figure 9.12.
The Upward Draw of Sexual Energy.

SEXUAL ENERGY CULTIVATION PRACTICES FOR MEN

Taoist masters discovered some five thousand years ago that after a man ejaculates, his chi becomes depleted and needs to be replenished. They identified excessive ejaculation as the primary reason for premature aging, sickness, and physical weakness in men. Taoists suggest that men apply the Golden Rule, which means the older a man gets, the more he needs to be mindful about preserving his energy by controlling his ejaculation.

THE GOLDEN RULE FOR MEN

AGE	DAYS BETWEEN EJACULATIONS
20	4
30	8
40	16
50	21
60	30+

Today we know that the testicles are amazing biological factories that produce several million sperm every day, and about 1,500 sperm every second. Each ejaculation releases from 15 to 200 million sperm per milliliter of semen. Spermatogenesis uses up to three hundred proteins and takes up to sixty days to restock a man's semen after a single ejaculation. That's a lot of energy!

The Tao teaches that when a man ejaculates excessively, his body starts borrowing energy from its own life force and its emergency reserves of energy stored in the kidneys. This can leave many organs depleted, including the brain. And as we discussed earlier, the first organ to sacrifice itself for the sake of any other organ is the skin, which begins to slow down its rate of renewal and regeneration. Therefore any man who wants to have healthy and youthful skin needs to learn how to preserve his sexual energy. Taoists do not suggest suppressing one's natural urges. Instead, they teach a powerful practice for transforming semen back into the life force.

If you're new to these practices you may find some of them may fall outside of your comfort zone. That's okay. Try the exercises that feel right for you and skip the others. While doing all of the practices will bring the greatest benefit, even doing just one will make a difference. We've provided the following exercises for the sake of sharing the broadest range of knowledge from the Tao, but if they make you feel uncomfortable, simply skip ahead to the next chapter and focus on other exercises and practices provided in this book.

 ## Smiling into Your Sexual Organs

Focusing your consciousness like a beam of sunshine into your testicles and kidneys helps transform semen into life force energy. For men, the sexual organs activate first, and then the heart activates. To have healthy-looking and vibrant skin, men and women both need heart radiance, which for men especially goes hand-in-hand with the health and vibrancy of one's sexual energy.

1. Start with slow abdominal breathing (p. 84 and 218). Imagine every breath going all the way to the spine.
2. Exhale completely and hold your breath, focusing on the center of your brain, the Crystal Palace (see p. 159, figure 8.9 for an illustration of the location of the Crystal Palace).
3. Inhale a few slow, deep breaths into your third eye. Focus on the Crystal Palace. Imagine you are capturing violet light in the center of your brain.
4. Sit quietly and focus on your kidneys and testicles, sending them smiling, loving energy while imagining the sun shining on the surface of water and turning the water into steam. Then focus on your Tan Tien and imagine a fire burning there, below your navel. Finally, smile into your heart and feel the fire burning and radiating. Doing this for a few minutes every day will help the transformation.

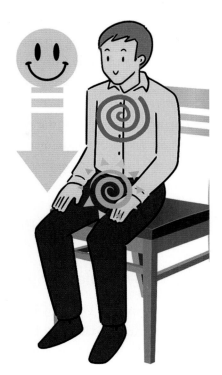

Figure 9.13. Smiling down into the sexual organs helps transform sexual energy stored there into chi.

 Testicle Massage

The testicles often develop energy blockages because of their complex blood circulation system. Many modern men spend long hours sitting, which interferes with the blood supply to the testicles. Restrictive clothing, excessive fat in the abdominal area, and a high level of stress are additional factors that contribute to energy blockages in the testicles. Therefore daily testicular massage is an essential practice. Testicular massage helps transform semen back into energy.

1. Warm your hands by rubbing them together. Then hold both testicles in your hands between your fingers and thumbs.
2. Pull your testicles downward until there is a very slight pain.
3. Massage your testicles with your fingers and thumbs, releasing the blockages. Release. Repeat nine times. The slight pain will lessen as the blockages are released.

4. Put one hand on your sacrum and another on the back of your head and feel chi moving up your spine.

5. Now sit and smile into your testicles, visualizing smiling sunshine on the surface of water, creating steam.

Taoists discovered that the space between the anus and the entire structure of the sexual organs in men is a powerful acupressure point. This point is considered so important that it has been called the "million dollar point." Massaging this point helps activate sexual energy flow and removes blockages. More information can be found in *Taoist Secrets of Love: Cultivating Male Sexual Energy* by Mantak Chia and Michael Winn.

Five-Minute Daily Chi Kung for Men

1. Knock on the Door of Life: Stand with your feet shoulder-width apart, the standard Chi Kung stance. Let your arms hang loosely by your sides. Turn your hips to the left and to the right, leading from your Tan Tian, and let your arms swing and loosely hit your abdomen and kidney area. This exercise activates your kidney fire.

2. Rotate your hips and your sacrum bone: Standing in the same posture, place both palms over your sacrum/kidney area on your back, and first make nine large circles with your hips in one direction, and then nine circles in the reverse direction. Then put one hand on your pubic bone while keeping the other hand on your sacrum and draw nine smaller circles in one direction with your tailbone only, and nine in the reverse direction. This exercise brings more blood and energy to the sexual organs and helps release blockages.

3. Tighten and release: Stand and focus on your perineum, located between your anus and your sexual organs. Smile and inhale as you simultaneously rise up to stand on your toes, roll your eyes up, clench your fists and jaws, and tighten your perineum. Then release, exhale, and return to the starting position. Repeat nine times. (You are going to use the same process when you do the Orgasmic Upward Draw, the practice described below.)

4. Close: Hold your kidneys with your palms, smile into your kidneys and sexual organs, and think of a fire burning in your kidney area.

Testicular Breathing (Cold Draw)

1. Stand and become aware of your testicles.
2. Inhale while imagining breathing into your testicles. Imagine your testicles expanding and contracting with every breath.
3. When you feel warmth, guide your energy with your breath from your testicles to your kidneys. This technique helps transform physical semen into energy, which then can be returned to the kidneys.

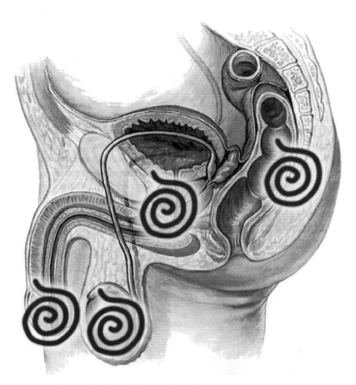

Figure 9.14. Chi moving throughout the male reproductive organs.

Male Orgasmic Upward Draw

Taoists have long known that sexuality is as important to our overall well-being as nutrition and exercise. Orgasm is not simply a momentary release, but a life-giving part of our overall health and longevity. By mastering mindfulness in orgasm and learning to retain the energy by transforming it back into chi, a man can ensure that not only his skin, but every organ in his body, including his brain, will have abundant chi for healing and regeneration. The Orgasmic Upward Draw for men is a technique that allows a man to retain his semen during orgasm in order to eventually transform it back into life-force energy.

1. On a scale 1 to 10, with 10 being closest to orgasm and ejaculation, bring yourself (on your own or with a partner) to a point from 7 to 8. At this point you are feeling an orgasm coming on but can still control the energy.
2. Next, stop, curl your toes, clench your fists, clench your jaws, roll your eyes up, pull up your perineum, and pull the orgasmic energy with your breath up your spine through the Microcosmic Orbit.

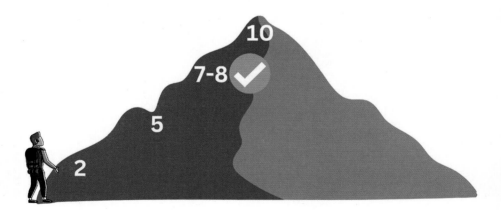

Figure 9.15. A man has to learn to recognize when he has reached the point of 7–8 on the 1–10 scale of orgasm.

Note: If you missed the 7–8 point, the Tao says you have reached the point of no return and it is very likely you won't be able to control your energy. The Tao calls this "overcooking your medicine." Be more careful next time! With practice you will be able to direct your orgasmic energy into your brain and then down through the Microcosmic Orbit, or wrap it around your kidneys to replenish your life force energy there. In this way your skin, as well as the rest of your organs, will always have enough energy for daily regeneration.

These practices have been used by generations of male and female practitioners of the Tao. In the higher spiritual practices of Taoism, a strong pelvic floor becomes the "chi muscle" or "spiritual muscle" that draws energy into the body. By supporting the pelvic floor, it is believed that we also support all the internal organs and prevent them from sagging. A strong pelvic floor, vibrant flow of sexual energy, and reduced anxiety and stress will increase confidence, creativity, and sexual magnetism at any age. Beautiful skin is just a bonus that results from the positive effects of sexual energy cultivation practices.

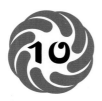

Iron Shirt Chi Kung to Maintain Strength and Beauty

Just as the skin is composed of many layers, so the whole body can be envisioned as layers of tissue. The outermost layer is the skin, the layer visible to ourself and to others. The second layer under that consists of subcutaneous fat, which is not visible to others, yet it defines (and sometimes distorts) the contours of the body and provides structural support and insulation. The next layer consists of muscles that are wrapped in a layer of connective tissue, or fascia. Muscles are attached to the bones, which provide structure and support for the body. Then there are the body's cavities that hold our internal organs, such as the heart, lungs, digestive system, brain, and sexual organs. Every organ in every cavity and the cavities themselves are lined in a layer of fascia, and it is this layer of fascia that ancient Taoist masters found could be packed with chi to support the internal organs and thereby supply radiant energy to the skin.

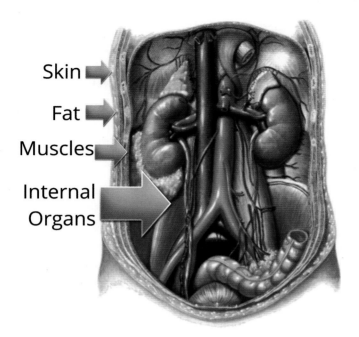

Skin

Fat

Muscles

Internal
Organs

Figure 10.1. The layers of the body: skin, fat (which is not limited to skin and is located just below the dermis), muscles (wrapped in fascia), bones (not shown), and internal organs.

FASCIA, THE BEST-KEPT SECRET OF RADIANCE

Many people do not realize how much their physical appearance depends on the health and strength of their fascia, bones, and muscles. The bones and muscles define facial and body contours, ensure alignment of soft tissues, and provide support for the skin. Fascia is rich in collagen and glycosaminoglycans, a family of polysaccharides that attracts water, which the body uses as a lubricant to provide elastic support and electrical conductivity throughout the body. When people age, the changes in their face and body result not only from changes in the skin and subcutaneous fat layer, but also from the slow deterioration and deformation of the bones, a weakening of the muscles, and a drying up and stiffening of the fascia.

To understand the importance of fascia, imagine taking an egg and dropping it on the ground. The egg will of course break. But if we put the egg inside an inflated balloon and then drop it on the ground, it has a much better chance of surviving the impact. If we take another balloon and put the first balloon with the egg inside it into that balloon, and even another, we will certainly be able to drop the egg on the ground without breaking it. In the same way, the chi inside the fascia works like air inside a balloon, protecting and uplifting the organs. In the past, martial artists learned to train in a special way in order to pack chi into their fascia. As a result, even a direct blow to the body would not damage their vital organs. Now most people do not have to worry about protecting their internal organs from heavy punches, but knowledge about how to build chi inside the fascia is very important when it comes to preserving the beauty and vitality of the skin, as well as the entire body.

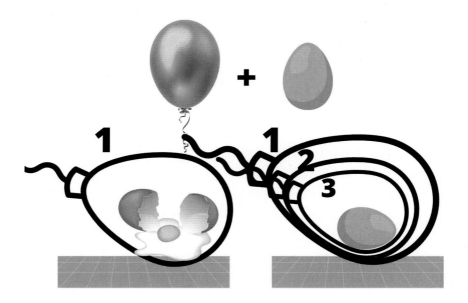

Figure 10.2. Egg inside three balloons experiment. Chi inside the fascia works like air inside a balloon, protecting and uplifting the organs.

When people age, their body starts sagging and slowly collapsing. This affects their internal organs, which have less space and less nourishment. When the internal organs are affected, the skin will be affected too, since its health and vitality depend on the health and vitality of the internal organs. When the fascia is filled with chi, it spreads to the bones and muscles and radiates throughout the skin, creating a youthful, vibrant glow.

The fascia has to be well-hydrated to function well. Since it's not so easy to move the blood inside fascia layers, physical movement is crucial. Without movement, the fascia will receive less and less hydration while also accumulating toxins and metabolic wastes.

An important organ made out of connective tissue is the mesentery (see also chapter 8). The mesentery is a thick membrane that contains

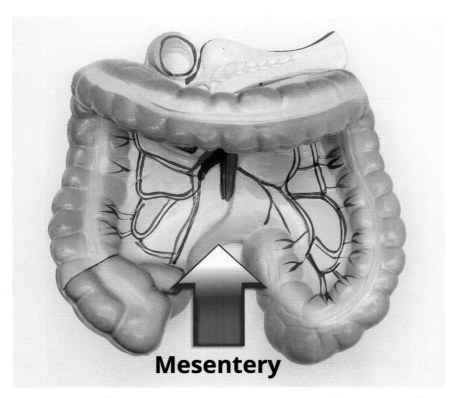

Mesentery

Figure 10.3. The mesentery, an organ that connects all the organs in the abdominal cavity together, is located in the Lower Tan Tien.

blood vessels, nerve fibers, and lymphatic vessels and connects all the organs in the abdominal cavity together. In the past it was believed that the mesentery was not an organ, but merely a membrane supporting the intestines, so surgeons did not hesitate to cut through it and remove parts of it. Now we know it to be an essential part of the enteric nervous system, which helps control the inner workings of the organs. Many Chi Kung exercises help bring more blood, oxygen, and nutrition to this structure to remove the toxins that can accumulate in it. Techniques such as abdominal breathing (p. 84 and 218) and Stem Cell Chi Kung (p. 108) can help keep the abdominal organs and fascia hydrated and oxygenated.

Another structure that depends on the health and hydration of the fascia is the pelvic floor, which is composed of muscles and fascia and supports the organs in the pelvic cavity and the entire body.

The skin of the face has a very special muscle-fascia layer known as the *superficial musculoaponeurotic system,* or SMAS, an area of musculature in the face that is interwoven into a continuous layer of fascia, which creates a kind of a moving mask. The facial muscles are not connected to

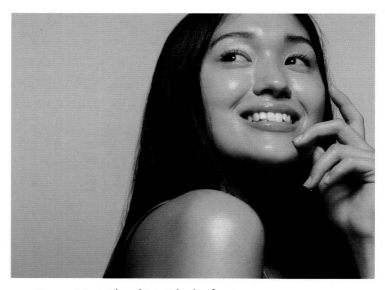

Figure 10.4. The chi inside the fascia can create a more uplifted facial expression.

the bones, but instead are attached to this fascial layer. This is why facial skin tends to sag and move downward with age. It's why skin stretches when people smile, laugh, cry, and make faces. Learning to pack more chi into the fascia and take care of the hydration and detox of not just the skin but the fascia as well can help create a more uplifted and younger-looking face.

Most Westerners who want to age well focus on exercises that build muscles. Ancient Taoists discovered that it is the fascia, as well as the joints and ligaments, that determines how youthful, agile, and energetic a person looks, feels, and performs as they get older.

Joints are structures that connect the bones, allowing flexibility and movement. It's thanks to the joints and ligaments that we don't walk like robots but instead can sway, sashay, bend, and turn. It is very important to realize that the joints need to be filled with lubricant liquid. This liquid is replenished, detoxed, and rejuvenated with tissue water, which is pushed into the joints when they move. The joints need to move in order to be soft, fluid, and flexible. If you sit too long and don't move, your joints cannot replenish their lubricant liquid—and it's impossible to be alluring, sexy, and confident if you have swollen, creaky, stiff joints.

BEAUTIFUL BONES

Taoist masters developed powerful techniques for enhancing bone and muscle strength to keep the body beautifully aligned and supported. Even in advanced age, Taoist sages have long demonstrated youthful agility and endurance, great posture, and swift, graceful movements. Modern science now confirms that Chi Kung and Tai Chi create biologically younger bones and muscles.[1]

Children and young adults have strong muscles, resilient bones, and flexible joints. A young child climbs trees, rides a bicycle, and runs down a hill with joy and abandon, without being concerned about falling. And even if the child falls, it rarely results in a broken bone. However for an older adult, any kind of fall can result in a fracture. The most common fractures in older adults are distal forearms, hips, and spine.[2] Every year, bone fragility in elderly people causes more than nine million fractures worldwide.[3] It is estimated that one in three women and one in five men over the age of fifty will suffer a fracture resulting from osteoporosis.

Physicians may recommend calcium supplements and exercises to support bone and muscle health, yet many healthy adults who exercise and eat wholesome food still suffer from fragile bones and weak muscle tissue. After reaching its peak in early adulthood, bone and muscle strength remains relatively constant unless a person makes an effort to exercise and develop both muscle and bone strength. However after age fifty, in both men and women, muscle mass starts declining at a rate of 1 to 2 percent per year, while muscle strength decreases at a rate of 1.5 to 3 percent per year. In eighty-year-old adults, there is an estimated 30 percent reduction in muscle mass and a 20 percent reduction in muscle area compared to twenty-year-olds.[4] Bone loss can start occurring as early as the age of thirty-five in both sexes, but accelerates in premenopausal women.[5]

Composition of the Bones

- **Osteoblasts:** short-lived bone-forming cells
- **Osteoclasts:** cells whose job it is to dissolve and resorb old or damaged bone tisssue
- **Osteocytes:** mature bone cells that can no longer differentiate
- **Bone marrow cells:** "blood cell factories"; they generate blood cells which are released into the bloodstream when matured and when needed
- **Fat cells:** create cushioning for bone marrow cells, participate in energy metabolism, and produce important growth factors

Bone marrow contains the precursors of blood cells. Bone marrow also contains a variety of stem cells and stemlike cells, including pluripotent mesenchymal stem cells that produce bone cells, cartilage, and fat; human skeletal stem cells that differentiate into bone and cartilage (but not fat); and periosteal stem cells, the main cells that repair the bone after damage. Hence bone tissue contains a rich pool of stem cells that when activated can heal fractures and restore bone tissue density and strength. One reason young people and children have strong and resilient bones is because they are able to remodel their bone structure quickly; they can destroy and remove old and damaged structures and replace them with new structures. As osteoclasts dissolve old boney tissue, the stem cells activate and start to differentiate into osteoblasts and then osteocytes (and, if needed, into cartilage and fat), replacing damaged structures. With age, less and less new bone is laid down and more and more microdamage accumulates. The goal, therefore, is to create the most favorable environment for bone and muscle growth and regeneration.

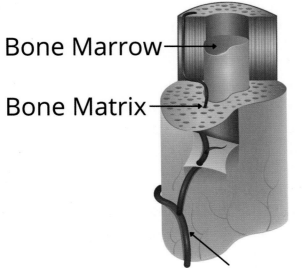

Figure 10.5. Inner structure of a bone.

FACTORS INFLUENCING BONE HEALTH

Like the skin, the bones can regenerate and heal. Even at an advanced age the bones and muscles never lose their ability to regenerate and grow, yet this capability is often greatly reduced. Several factors have been found to be essential for maintaining bone and muscle health:

- **Gravity and physical activity:** Scientific studies of physiological changes in astronauts who spend prolonged periods of time in space as well as studies of immobilized patients in hospitals demonstrate that both gravity and muscle activity are essential for proper bone growth.[6] It has been firmly established that at first the muscles start losing their strength, and then their mass starts wasting away. Lack of physical activity results in accelerated bone and muscle loss, while physical exercises help maintain strong bones and muscles.[7] Balanced activity is more beneficial to bone and muscle health than strenuous, repetitive physical tasks such as heavy lifting. Practices of Chi Kung include mindful alignment of the inner structure with the forces of gravity, as well as slow, mindful movements that create favorable conditions for bone growth.[8]

- **Hormonal changes:** After fifty, women have a higher risk of fractures and loss of muscle mass compared to men. Because estrogen has a protective effect on bone and muscle health, a deficiency later in life leads to increased risk of osteoporosis. For men, low testosterone is linked to weakening of the muscles. Testosterone levels gradually decrease in older men at a rate of 1 percent a year. Men who continue being physically active as they age can maintain strong muscles and bones despite this decrease in testosterone.

- **Effects of cigarette smoking, alcohol, and diet:** Smoking negatively impacts bone health and increases the risk of fractures. It is especially detrimental for women because the chemical compounds in cigarette smoke accelerate the breakdown of circulating estrogen, weakening the bones. Similarly, high alcohol intake increases the risk of fractures. There is no significant increase of risk, however, for people who limit their intake of alcohol to two or fewer drinks a day.

- **Weight:** Many women over fifty start experiencing weight gain and try to address it with dieting and strenuous exercise. However studies suggest that being thin and lean may actually increase the risk of fractures in perimenopausal women. It is, however, important to notice that the relationship between body weight and the risk of fractures is complex, and both low body weight and obesity may increase the risk of fractures through different mechanisms.[9] One explanation is that after menopause, most of the estrogen in the blood comes from fatty tissue, which converts androgen into estrogen. Carrying a little bit of extra weight actually ensures a sufficient level of estrogen to maintain bone health. As well, those who have a heavier body put more weight on their bones, activating their adaptive regeneration. It is also possible that the reason for the reduced risk of fractures in slightly overweight women may be the protective cushioning provided by that extra weight.[10]

- **Inflammation and glucocorticoids:** Both inflammation and the use of anti-inflammatory oral glucocorticoids, also known as steroids, result in an increased risk of osteoporosis and fractures. Bone loss caused by steroids is more noticeable in the first month of treatment and is most significant in the spine. Rheumatoid arthritis and ankylosing spondylitis (a type of arthritis that causes inflammation of the bones and ligaments of the spine) increase the risk of osteoporosis and fractures due to both limited mobility and inflammation. The Longitudinal Aging Study of Amsterdam demonstrated that high levels of the cytokine interleukin 6 (IL-6) are linked to loss of muscle mass. One explanation is that low-grade chronic inflammation suppresses regeneration and accelerates tissue breakdown.[11]

- **Chemical "crosstalk":** Until recently it was believed that the bones provide mechanical structural support for the muscles and are moved by the pulling and twisting force of the muscles, and that they are not metabolically active tissue. It is now established, however, that not only do the muscles secrete biologically active messengers that regulate metabolism, so do the bone cells, the osteocytes, which act as endocrine cells, producing compounds that affect the muscles and other organs such as the kidneys. Today it is widely accepted that the bones and muscles "talk" through a host of chemical messengers. This explains why physical exercise is so important for maintaining bone and muscle health. It also explains why inflammation, which creates a biochemically different microenvironment, has a negative effect on the bones and muscles. Chemical messengers secreted by the bones can influence the muscles in the skin and accelerate aging. Psychological stress and perpetual worry increase inflammation throughout the body, including the bones and muscles.[12]

TAOIST CHI KUNG FOR STRUCTURE AND SUPPORT

Taoist masters traditionally devoted great care to maintaining one's body structure. They held that bones work like crystals that can condense and transmit radiant energy. They used bones to receive chi from the universe and to store chi. By condensing chi in the bones, the bone structure becomes stronger and better resists the decline that comes with aging. Because bones work like crystals, accumulating radiant chi in your bones helps increase your inner radiance, allowing you to project it outward. Special exercises such as a form of Taoist yoga called Tao Yin, Tai Chi, as well as the abbreviated Iron Shirt Chi Kung practice found in this chapter have been developed to make the bones strong and to help accumulate radiant energy in the bones. The same techniques can be used to ensure preservation of facial contour, good posture, and overall radiance.

Taoist practices to strengthen the bones begin with establishing one's rootedness in Mother Earth. According to the Tao, connection to earth energy is the most important practice to master on the physical plane. The practices of Iron Shirt Chi Kung became especially popular among martial artists in China. Since Kung Fu fighters must have a stable posture and must be able to endure heavy blows to their bodies, developing strength of the bones and protective powers of the muscles and fascia was a life-saving skill. For modern women and men who want to have naturally smooth, resilient, radiant skin, Iron Shirt practices provide a path to using the uplifting and supportive power of chi to counteract sagging caused by gravity.

Many people develop chronic anxiety as they get older, which leads to tension in the rib cage. In the Taoist tradition it is believed that the boney structures in the chest are affected by the energy of the heart. When the heart is full of negative emotions, especially hatred, it can leak into the bones and accumulate in the rib cage and sternum. Taoists believe that resentment, grudges, and hatred can turn the bones black. Modern

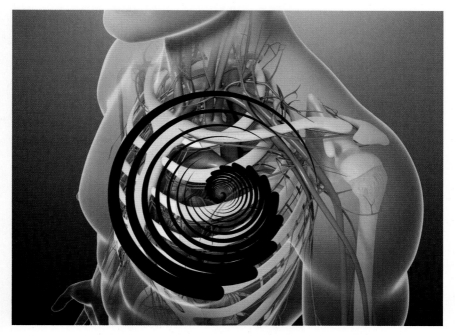

Figure 10.6. Negative energy in the heart can affect the bones of the rib cage.

science confirms that anxiety and tension in the muscles can affect the bones by impeding blood flow and creating chronic inflammation.[13]

Taoists place great importance on all the bones, especially those that form the spine, because without it the body would collapse in a pile of flesh and bones. One bone that receives special attention in the Taoist tradition is the sacrum, which is a flat, sturdy bone at the base of the spine that has eight holes through which nerves from the spinal cord enter the pelvic area. Nowadays, many people spend a lot of time sitting down, and this affects blood flow in the sacral area. This in turn affects the vitality of all the pelvic organs, including the sexual organs. In the Taoist tradition, the sacrum is considered one of the most important pumps, helping move chi and spinal fluid up the spine. The sacral pump works in tandem with the cranial pump at the base of the skull.

Most people never think of their bones as something that can breathe, feed, regenerate, and rejuvenate. However bones are living tissues and they receive up to 10 percent of the total blood volume pumped by the heart with every heartbeat. Bones receive oxygen, nutrients, and

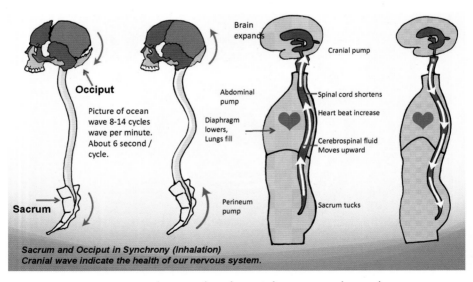

Figure 10.7. The sacral and cranial pumps work together
to move spinal fluid and chi.

chemical growth factors, and just like any other tissue they have to get rid of metabolic wastes, CO_2, and acid. Unlike cartilage, which does not have cells or blood vessels, the bones are alive and can regenerate. They also can grow old, brittle, and dry. Blood flows into the bones through nutrient arteries that enter the inner cavities of the bones. Then the blood travels through the sinuses of the bone marrow and numerous tiny capillaries that deliver blood, oxygen, nutrients, and regulatory molecules into the cortex, where baby bone cells can feed and grow. As people grow older, the blood supply to the bones declines, causing the bones to become drier, with less developed bone marrow and less active stem cells. As the bones' inner environment becomes more suffocating and acidic, the bones activate special cells called *osteoclasts,* which start dissolving and digesting the bones, making them weak and easily deformed. It's not easy for the heart to push blood through all the bones in the body. Taoist masters discovered that it is possible, however, to improve blood flow through the bones by means of exercises that turn large muscles into additional "hearts" that can help the main heart muscle move blood through the body (fig. 10.8, p. 214).

The bone marrow is where red blood cells and the cells of the immune system develop and grow. When blood flow to the inner bones declines with age, it negatively affects formation of blood cells and immunity. The percentage of marrow space occupied by hematopoietic tissue goes from a high of 40 to 60 percent in young adults to just 20 to 40 percent in older people. The rest of that space is taken up by fat. The body will never run out of blood because of declining bone marrow, but it will have to spend much more energy manufacturing the same amount of blood cells from a much lower number of stem cells.

Bones change so slowly that most people fail to notice when and how their face became longer, their eyes started looking hollow, their chin moved, and their body developed the slumped posture of an old person. No matter what cosmetic product a person uses, their bones reveal their true age. Bones are heavy. When people are constantly grumpy, sad, and depressed, their muscles pull the bones down. In the Tao it is believed that heavy and toxic emotional energy can accumulate

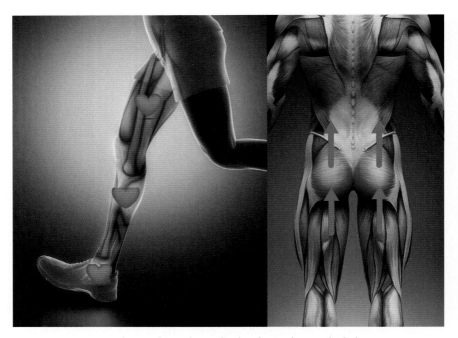

Figure 10.8. Muscles in the calves, thighs, buttocks, and abdomen serve as extra "hearts" to help the heart pump blood.

in the bones. When everything pulls the bones down and nothing lifts them up, the face will eventually become longer. Bone resorption and loss of gum tissue may alter the chin area, pushing the chin back. As bones move down and become thinner, the orbital rim becomes more spacious, and this deepens the hollows under the eyes. Bones do take a long time to change, but once they start changing it is extremely difficult to reverse the changes. Chi Kung practices help make the bones lighter by creating uplifting energy in the body and by releasing heavy, toxic energy.

MUSCLES AND MOVEMENT

The dangers of osteoporosis are well-known. Less well-known is sarcopenia, the gradual loss of muscle mass and strength, which can greatly increase the risk of fractures by affecting posture, balance, and bone strength. It is now confirmed that the bones respond to mechanical signals from the muscles and adapt their growth and regeneration to support physical demands. A 2009 sarcopenia and hip fracture study[14] of 193 subjects who had suffered previous minimal trauma hip fractures found that in the year following the initial hip fracture, 75 percent of subjects had reduced muscle mass, 56 percent fell at least once, 28 percent had multiple falls, 12 percent had a new fracture affecting a different bone, and 5 percent had another hip fracture.

Muscles support bone structures and further define body shape. In athletic people, well-developed muscles define the shape of the body, the effects of which contribute to one's self-image and personal confidence. The facial muscles as well as other muscles in the body influence the skin's health and beauty. For example, the chest muscles and diaphragm participate in breathing, which is essential for energy production. The diaphragm is a big muscle. If someone is constantly stressed and has a lot

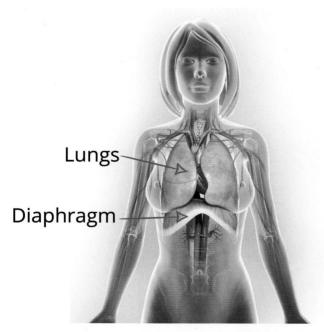

Figure 10.9. The chest muscles and diaphragm are involved in breathing. It is very difficult to be beautiful and radiant if your breathing is restricted.

of anxiety, their diaphragm will get tense and their breathing becomes shallow, which affects energy production. It is very difficult to be beautiful and radiant if your breathing is restricted. This is one of the many reasons why anxiety and stress are so detrimental to beauty.

Another important muscle to pay attention to is the psoas, a long lateral muscle located in the lateral lumbar region between the vertebral column and the brim of the lesser pelvis that allows us to maintain an upright posture. When this muscle weakens, it results in a bent spine, shuffling feet, and an unsteady gait. Taoists believe that the psoas muscle is a spiritual muscle, and its maintenance and development is essential for one's spiritual growth.

Thousands of years ago, Taoists discovered something that science has discovered only recently. By moving the body regularly we can not only reverse age-related muscle loss, we can also restore our bones to health. Various studies show that physical exercise can rejuvenate the DNA so that it starts producing proteins similar to those of a younger body.[15] Taoist Chi Kung practices include moving meditations that train not only the muscles and bones, but also the mind. Muscles can regenerate faster than bones. It still takes time to repair a muscle or build a stronger muscle, but it can be done faster than growing a new bone. By increasing

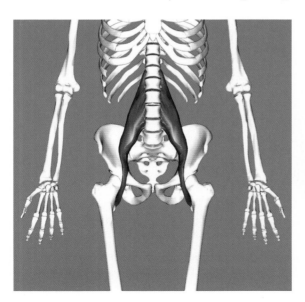

Figure 10.10.
The psoas muscle, found on both sides of the vertebral column, holds the body upright and defines posture.

muscle strength, we can help the bones stay younger, which helps us resist age-related changes. By packing chi inside the fascia and bones, we can ensure that the skin will remain uplifted, radiant, and vital.

INTRODUCTION TO IRON SHIRT CHI KUNG

Age should not be an obstacle to having a body that moves with ease, with a well-aligned and beautiful posture. When the bones and muscles are aligned, the skin has more support and displays fewer signs of sagging and wrinkling. Even wrinkles look more beautiful when the skin has good support and its natural radiance comes through. Iron Shirt Chi Kung is a Taoist practice that uses mindful breathing and aligned posture to strengthen the internal organs, clean out toxins, and help convert fat stored in the body into chi so that it can be used to fortify the fascia, the bones, and the entire body. During this practice we pack chi into the fascia so that it provides better support for the bones and ligaments, aligning the entire body into a smoothly and gracefully moving system. Another advantage of this practice is improved breathing and circulation. This too helps detox and energize the body and skin.

Before doing the Iron Shirt practices it is important to practice Inner Smile Chi Kung as described in chapter 4, the Six Healing Sounds meditation found in chapter 7, and the Microcosmic Orbit practice found in chapter 8. This will ensure that you are relaxed, smiling, and have a cleaner, fresher chi in your body and minimal toxic emotional energy. It is beneficial to practice the Inner Smile while standing in the Iron Shirt posture. The complete practice of Iron Shirt Chi Kung is beyond the scope of this book, so here we are giving you just the basics. For the complete practice, refer to Master Mantak Chia's book *Iron Shirt Chi Kung.*[16]

It is preferable, if possible, to find a certified Universal Healing Tao instructor to ensure that you do Iron Shirt Chi Kung correctly. This practice is not a substitute for qualified medical care and is not meant to treat any medical conditions. The following exercises will introduce you to the basics of the Iron Shirt and give you a road map for future study and practice.

Preparation 1: Abdominal Breathing

1. Stand in Chi Kung posture with your feet shoulder-width apart, your body relaxed and at ease, tailbone slightly tucked in, and shoulders relaxed.

2. Inhale, drawing air in and expanding your abdomen. Make sure you expand not only the front, but also the sides of your body, as if you were creating a belt around your midline. Focus on the feeling of lowering your diaphragm, creating a hollow feeling in the chest.

3. Hold your breath for a moment and then exhale and let your abdomen naturally flatten. Relax as you exhale.

4. Inhale again, dropping the diaphragm and allowing the abdomen to expand on all sides like a ball. Then pull your perineum and sexual organs up, holding pressure in the abdomen for a moment. Exhale, while continuing to pull your sexual organs up and your navel toward your spine.

5. Repeat the breathing pattern from step 4 nine times, with each inhalation and exhalation counted as one set. Later you can extend the repetitions to eighteen or thirty-six times. Make sure you are relaxed throughout this practice. There should be no pushing or forcing yourself.

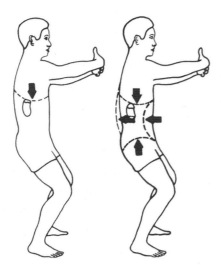

Figure 10.11. Movements of the diaphragm during abdominal breathing.

Preparation 2: Easy Chi-Packing Breathing

The following process of packing chi into the body is slow and easy. It is important to notice your body and listen to what it's telling you. Read the steps carefully to make sure you understand and can follow correctly.

1. Sit on the edge of a chair. Imagine a place in nature that is comforting and relaxing. Smile and relax.
2. Inhale, lowering your diaphragm and expanding your abdomen, keeping your focus on your Lower Tan Tien, the area just below your navel. Exhale and let your abdomen flatten as you keep your focus below your navel and pull your sexual organs up. Focus on the feeling of expansion and then a feeling of release as you inhale and exhale.
3. Continue to breathe in this pattern, making sure your breath is very slow and relaxed, focusing on smiling, relaxing, expanding, and releasing.

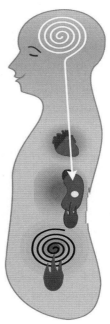

Figure 10.12. Guiding chi into the kidneys and lower abdomen.

4. When you are comfortable with keeping a mindful, relaxed, and smiling focus on your expansion and release, you can proceed to the next step.

5. Inhale and expand your abdomen. Pull your sexual organs and perineum up. Bring your attention to your left kidney. Slowly exhale, guiding chi with your eyes, your mind, and your breath into your left kidney. Rest and spiral chi in the kidney.

6. Inhale and expand your abdomen. Pull up your sexual organs and perineum. Bring your attention to your right kidney. Slowly and mindfully exhale, guiding chi with your eyes, your mind, and your breath into your right kidney. Rest and spiral chi into the kidney.

7. Inhale and expand your abdomen. Pull up your sexual organs and perineum. Bring your attention to your lower abdomen. Slowly exhale, guiding chi with your eyes, your mind, and your breath, into your lower abdomen. Rest and spiral chi in your lower abdomen.

8. Relax, focusing your attention below your navel.

Embrace the Tree Posture

This practice combines standing in an aligned and rooted posture with abdominal breathing and packing chi into the body. Rootedness is very important in the Taoist tradition, as Mother Earth's energy is essential for all spiritual growth. Since earth energy is creative and life-giving, it is very important to learn how to connect to earth's power and draw this energy from the feet upward.

1. Stand in Chi Kung posture with your feet shoulder-width apart, knees slightly bent. Turn your toes slightly inward for better stability. Make sure all your toes, the ball of your feet, the heels, and the edges of the feet are connecting to the ground.

2. Focus on the soft spots right below the bones of your toes, called the Bubbling Springs (see p. 161, figure 8.10 for an illustration of this point), and imagine them having an earthward suction. Imagine having deep roots growing from your feet into the ground.

3. Slightly bend your knees so that they are in a straight line above your toes. Do not let your knees go forward of your toes.

4. Slightly tuck your tailbone and relax your chest and shoulders. Imagine that you were about to sit down in a chair and then changed your mind. You can practice this position with your spine against the wall to ensure proper alignment.

5. Slowly raise your arms and hold them rounded them in front of you, chest-high, as if you were holding a large ball or embracing a large tree. Your collarbone and your arms should be linked together so that if you imagine a flow of energy circulating through your rounded arms it would pass through your collarbones. Spread your fingers slightly and keep your thumbs up. At first you will use your muscles to hold your arms up, but the more

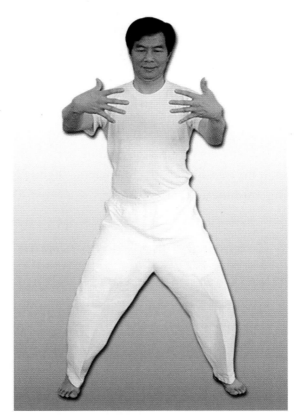

Figure 10.13.
Embrace the Tree posture.

chi you build, the more you will be able to relax and enjoy feeling the movement of chi.

6. Imagine that your head is suspended from the ceiling by an invisible thread. As the universal force pulls you up and gravity pulls you down, your spine will relax and elongate.

7. Start abdominal breathing as described in the exercise above. Take it easy and remember to smile and relax.

8. Use Easy Chi-Packing Breathing, described in the previous exercise, to guide chi you're your kidneys and lower abdomen. When you master the practice you will be able to pack chi into all the fascia in the abdominal cavity and, finally, into the fascia supporting your skin.

Standing in the Embrace the Tree posture is a calming meditation that aligns the body with gravitational forces. As you gradually restore the internal pressure of chi in the fascia layers you will notice a more uplifted, radiant, and vital appearance of the skin of not only the face, but the entire body. Taoists believe that earth has abundant healing energy that can be absorbed through the feet. Gradually you will learn to feel this energy and use it to replenish the body. You can enhance this meditation by imagining that you are a tree standing in the forest, feeling your roots spreading deeper and deeper into the ground, with your arms becoming like branches of the tree, filled with chi. Imagine slightly swaying in the wind, absorbing sunshine and earth energy.

Embrace the Tree in Nature

When you can stand in a relaxed and aligned posture for at least three to five minutes, you can practice this variation of the Iron Shirt Embrace the Tree meditation, especially if you have access to a forest, a park, or have a nature area in your backyard. This version combines the Iron Shirt, the Inner Smile, communing with a tree, and the Microcosmic Orbit.

1. Find a healthy young tree. Stand outside of the boundaries defined by its crown. Ground yourself and feel your feet growing roots connecting you to the ground.
2. Take a few deep, full breaths and smile at the tree. Mentally ask the tree for its permission to connect. If you feel the answer is no, find another tree. If you feel the answer is yes, proceed to the next step.
3. Take a step closer and now stand inside the inner circle of the tree as defined by its crown. Assume the Embrace the Tree posture (without actually touching the tree). Feel your feet connected to the earth, your spine elongated, and your tailbone tucked in. Imagine your head is suspended from above by a silk thread.
4. Smile at the tree and into your own body. Relax and breathe naturally. Now start running the Microcosmic Orbit, first through your own body and then through the trunk of the tree.
5. As you smile and relax, ask the tree to take your negative energy, which can be used for the growth and replenishment of the tree, and exchange it for vibrant and vital life force.
6. You can finish by guiding fresh, vibrant chi into your internal organs, fascia, skin, and bones. Finish by thanking the tree for sharing its gifts of chi with you.

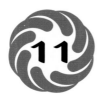

Common Skin Problems

The Tao teaches that both a deficiency and an excess of energy are unhealthy and can create problems. Deficiency of energy in the skin causes delayed regeneration, lack of radiance, and early aging. However, an excess of energy is equally damaging. One example of the damaging effects of excess energy is that caused by the sun's UV radiation. Since solar radiation is energy that affects the skin, both a deficiency and an excess of solar radiation create problems. When the skin receives enough sunshine it produces vitamin D_3, which is vital not only for skin, but for the entire body. Sunlight is known to help the skin produce endorphins, which elevate mood, alleviate pain, reduce inflammation, and heal and regenerate. However UV radiation can also damage collagen, elastin, and glycosaminoglycans in the skin, and disrupt the formation of new skin, leading to early wrinkling, pigment spots, and an uneven, coarse texture. In some cases, UV radiation may damage cells' proteins and DNA, creating the conditions for developing skin cancer.

Dermatologists are constantly advising us to use sunscreen to protect the skin from the deleterious effects of UV radiation. As well, many people either use sunscreen improperly so that it doesn't offer any real protection, or they care only about preventing sunburn while trying to get a beautiful tan, which defies the whole purpose of using a sunscreen. The Tao teaches that it is important to understand the nature of the energy we are dealing with in order to develop a suitable practice.

SUNLIGHT AND ITS EFFECTS

The sun emits fire energy, which is yang, meaning it's hot, expanding, and bright. Fire can be life-giving or it can burn and destroy life. This metaphor helps us understand the complex interaction between the skin and sunlight. UV radiation constitutes only 10 percent of the sunlight spectrum, but it is a very important part. It is defined as all light with a wavelength longer than X-rays and shorter than visible light. Infrared radiation, which is perceived as heat, has an even longer wavelength compared to visible light. We cannot see or feel UV radiation,

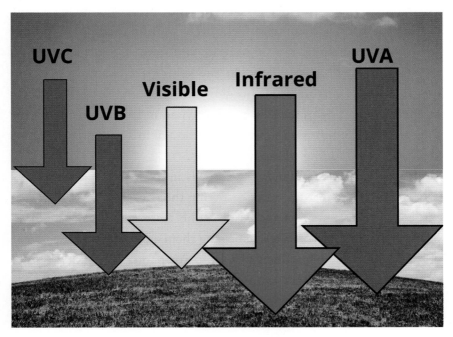

Figure 11.1. Types of light energy emitted by the sun: infrared radiation, visible light, UVA, UVB, UVC, and X-rays. Only infrared radiation, visible light, UVA, and UVB radiation reach the surface of Earth.

which makes it dangerous, because many of its most detrimental effects are delayed and only manifest years after the initial damage.

All UV radiation emitted by the sun is divided to three parts depending on the wavelength and effects. UVA radiation has a wavelength of 315–400 nanometers (nm). It is often referred to as "soft UV" and many people consider it safe. However, with prolonged exposure it can still damage the skin's proteins and DNA. Because UVA radiation produces a beautiful tan without sunburn, it is used in tanning salons, but it's important to remember that no UV radiation is completely safe. Next is UVB radiation, which is 280–315 nm and has a higher energy. It is partially absorbed by the ozone layer, so we get only a limited portion of it. This type of UV is responsible for tanning and burning. Finally, UVC is the shortest UV radiation, 100–280 nm, and it is extremely damaging to the skin, but fortunately it is completely absorbed by Earth's ozone layer.

The sun's effects on the skin can be immediate and delayed. First, the skin feels warm and nice because sunshine brings life-giving energy to the skin. Brief exposure to sunlight in the morning hours can improve one's mood by helping the skin release endorphins. Since endorphins relax and open deep capillaries in the skin, brief exposure to warm sunshine helps create a beautiful glow and radiance. It also improves regeneration and helps the skin produce vitamin D. This would be the equivalent of the morning sun warming the soil in a garden, nourishing the flowers and adding vibrancy to colors.

If sun exposure continues beyond this initial warm and welcoming interaction, UV radiation starts triggering the release of free radicals of oxygen from the skin's proteins. These highly reactive molecules can react with the skin's lipid structures, damaging them and triggering the release of the highly toxic byproducts of lipid peroxidation. The skin's surface contains antioxidants that can neutralize free radicals and prevent the skin's lipids from "catching on fire" from lipid peroxidation. If, however, a person continues exposing their skin to the sun's ultraviolet light, its antioxidant system will eventually become overwhelmed. One way to help the skin stay safe under the sun is to supplement it with skin-care products containing natural antioxidants or nutrition rich in antioxidants.[1]

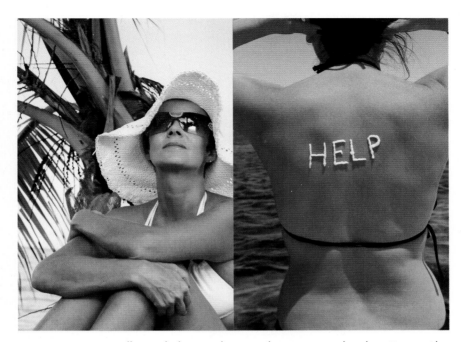

Figure 11.2. Initially, sunlight stimulates and invigorates the skin. Too much sunshine, however, damages the skin.

Probably everyone has had a sunburn at least once in their lifetime. Even though sunburn is unpleasant, it is nevertheless the first line of skin defense against UV-induced damage, because it activates a process known as programmed cell death, or apoptosis, during which damaged skin cells are destroyed before they cause any further problems. However it is accompanied by inflammation and oxidative stress, which by itself can cause skin damage.[2] But with the advent of modern sunscreens, sunburn has become rarer. This may be not a good thing, though, because without the familiar risk of sunburn, we may tend to spend too much time exposing our skin to the sun.[3] This was especially dangerous in the past, when most sunscreens protected the skin only from UVB radiation, the kind that causes the skin to burn and blister, but did not protect against UVA radiation, which causes the desired suntan.[4] One way to see the difference between natural skin aging and sun-induced premature aging is to compare the skin on exposed areas such as the face, décolleté, hands, arms, and legs, with areas of skin that are mostly hidden from the sun, such as the inside of the thighs.[5]

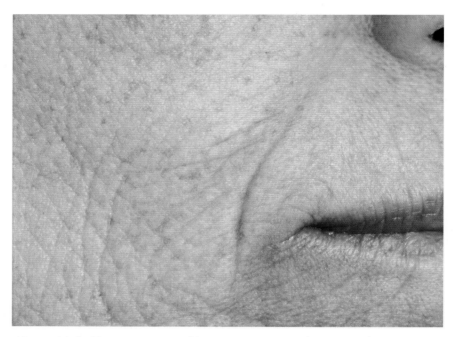

Figure 11.3. Skin aging caused by excessive UV radiation produces coarse, deep wrinkles and pigment spots.

One of many problems associated with sunscreens is that some UV filters, which consist of chemicals used to protect the skin from the damaging effects of UV radiation, release a mixture of free radicals and other toxic compounds into the skin if a person spends too much time exposed to solar radiation. However no matter how many times people hear that they should not try to get a tan and that they'll be better off protecting their skin and staying in the shade, the allure of tanned skin is just too strong.

The truth is that UV radiation is a constantly present damaging factor. The sun is a blazing nuclear reactor in the sky that emits powerful waves of electromagnetic radiation. Thankfully most of it is absorbed or blocked by our atmosphere, but even the small portion that reaches Earth is enough to cause damage to biological structures, including the skin. Every living organism on Earth has many levels of protection against the damaging effects of UV radiation, including antioxidants, natural UV filters, and various surface coverings such as slime, wax, shells, scales, fur, and feathers. Only human beings knowingly expose their unprotected naked skin to hot, burning sunlight in order to obtain a fashionable tan. Even now, with all the scientific evidence, many people still find it hard to believe that the common practice of tanning, which requires excessive exposure to sunlight, leads to premature wrinkling, withered skin, pigment spots, and in some cases, skin cancer.

Since human skin is not protected by fur or feathers, its only protection is the thin layer of cornified cells on its surface, skin oil, the antioxidant system, and a special pigment called *melanin.* Therefore a tan is not a fashion statement, but a protective reaction. Melanin has a dual function. First, it absorbs UV radiation, preventing it from reaching skin cells. Also, in the process of melanin synthesis there are many intermediate products that have protective and antioxidant properties. The very fact that nature invented such a complex mechanism to keep

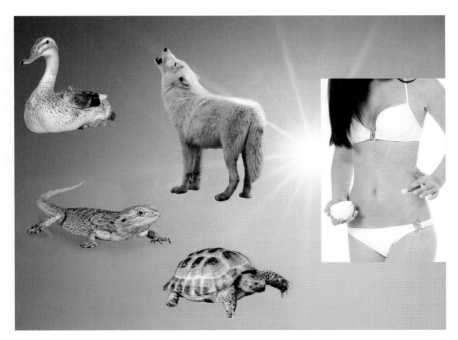

Figure 11.4. Animals protect their skin from UV radiation with shells, scales, slime, fur, and feathers. Humans have only their clothing and sunscreens.

UV radiation from reaching the skin cells should be enough to demonstrate the very real dangers of UV radiation on the skin.

Different types of skin have different abilities to produce melanin. For example, the skin of red-headed people does not tan well because it contains a different kind of melanin, pheomelanin, which tends to accumulate in freckles, providing very poor protection.[6] Most people have some combination of pheomelanin and eumelanin (the one which is found in sun tanned and naturally black and brown skin). Eumelanin is photoprotective with SPF around 3–4. It works as a broad-spectrum sunscreen, while its precursors have antioxidant properties.

Naturally black and brown skin has a higher density of melanin which is more evenly distributed and therefore it is considered better protected from UV-induced damage. However, it also can be damaged and needs protection from excessive UV exposure.[7] Skin of any color is more beautiful when it is healthy and radiant, so anything that throws the skin out of balance is neither beautiful nor healthy.

All cells in the skin, including the ones that make hair follicles, sebaceous glands, and sweat glands, are affected by the sun and stress, causing such common disorders as hair loss, dandruff, acne, and increased skin oiliness. Another skin condition strongly affected by stress is psoriasis. Interestingly, all inflammatory skin conditions, including psoriasis, are improved by moderate sun exposure, but excessive sun exposure, especially when combined with stress, is very detrimental. One of the molecules responsible for the beneficial effects of moderate sun exposure is nitric oxide. It is a small, ubiquitous molecule that triggers the relaxation of the blood vessels, lowers blood pressure, and increases circulation. Nitric oxide is also involved in cell growth and repair. When the skin is exposed to sunlight, its cells release nitric oxide, which in turn stimulates the release of endorphins. This reaction is responsible for the feeling of pleasure and relaxation associated with sunlight. However, with prolonged exposure, these beneficial effects are outweighed by the detrimental effects inflicted by free radicals and inflammation. As the Tao constantly reminds us, balance is key.

Currently, dermatologists recommend exposing the skin to sunlight for ten to fifteen minutes daily, in the morning hours. One should avoid sunbathing between 11 a.m. and 2 p.m. A sunscreen should be used to protect the skin from excessive UV exposure, but not to extend your time on the beach in order to get a better tan.

Just as fire provides warmth and comfort when it is contained but can burn down houses and whole forests when it is out of control, sunshine should be used in moderation. Just as the sun can give life to a garden, it can also dry the soil and vegetation; similarly, sunshine can improve circulation, boost immunity, release endorphins, and repair the skin, or it can trigger the release of harmful free radicals, increase inflammation, and destroy collagen and elastin, causing premature aging and pigment spots. Moreover, when combined with stress, UV radiation is especially dangerous for aging skin. Taoist practices such as the

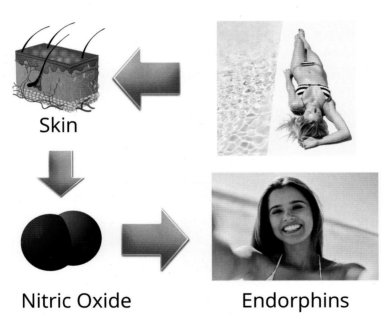

Skin

Nitric Oxide   Endorphins

Figure 11.5. Sunlight in moderation triggers nitric oxide in the skin, which triggers endorphins, resulting in a feeling of relaxation and pleasure and producing a beautiful glow, allowing the skin to repair itself.

Inner Smile (chapter 4) and the Six Healing Sounds (chapter 7) balance the emotions, release stress, and increase the production of beneficial neurochemicals.

DARK CIRCLES UNDER THE EYES AND PIGMENT SPOTS

One of the most common signs of stress and lack of sleep is the appearance of dark circles under the eyes. It's a condition that instantly makes people look visibly aged and unhealthy.

The skin is a complex and highly active organ that produces and responds to a multitude of neurotransmitters, hormones, and other messengers. In particular, it synthetizes chemicals involved in the hypothalamus-pituitary-adrenal (HPA) axis, which is the system of communication between the hypothalamus and the pituitary gland in the brain and the adrenal glands in the kidneys. Now we know that this system includes chemical and neurological connections between the brain, the gut, and the skin. Because of this interconnectedness, the skin is affected not only

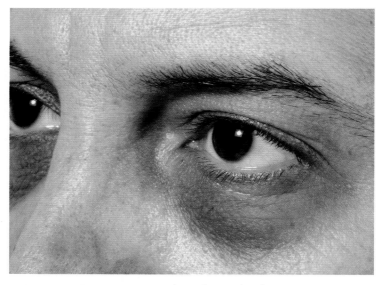

Figure 11.6. Dark circles under the eyes.

by environmental factors such as pollution and UV radiation, but also by emotional stress. Among the chemicals involved in the stress response, the major ones are the corticosteroids, and in particular, cortisol.

Skin cells have receptors to cortisol, so every time cortisol is elevated, the skin is affected. Prolonged exposure to glucocorticoids, both natural and those found in prescription medications, slows down skin repair, impairing its barrier function and immunity. Studies have demonstrated that when excessive UV exposure is combined with stress, it significantly increases the level of active cortisol in the skin. This leads to delayed wound healing, slowed-down collagen synthesis, and an increase in inflammation.[8] These effects increase with age. The same level of stress and the same amount of time spent getting a tan will be more detrimental to the skin after the age of fifty compared to skin before the age of twenty-five. The addition of cigarette smoking and pollution, combined with stress, sun exposure, and aging, increases the deterioration of the supporting collagen matrix in the skin, leading to wrinkles, skin sagging, and other changes. This is because stress, sun, cigarette smoke, and pollution all lead to the generation of damaging free radicals in the skin along with the depletion of its natural antioxidant system, an increase of inflammation, and the activation of enzymes that destroy the collagen and elastin structures in the skin.[9]

It turns out that dark circles under the eyes are due to the accumulation of pigments such as melanin and bilirubin, which have antioxidant and anti-inflammatory properties. When the skin is stressed and exposed to too much sun, it recruits additional systems to keep it safe. Ironically, the substances that come to the rescue also create uneven pigmentation. Nobody wants dark circles under their eyes. Nobody wants pigment spots on their skin. However this is nature's way of bringing attention to unhealthy conditions. Just as pain signals that something in the body requires our attention, pigment conditions such as dark under-eye circles and age spots indicate that the skin needs help. There are many skin-care products that help fade away dark circles and pigment spots. They may contain kojic acid, mulberry extract, hydroquinone, and other skin lighteners. They do not, however, resolve the underlying problem. Hydroquinone, a type of phenol commonly prescribed for removing pigment lesions, is particularly toxic to skin cells, so it may actually aggravate skin damage and accelerate aging. Another reason for dark circles under the eyes is oxidation of proteins by toxic free radicals. Many oxidized proteins change their color and appear dark when they accumulate in the skin.

It is well-established that "feel-good" molecules such as beta-endorphins and encephalin, released through smiling, relaxation, and mind-centered physical exercises such as yoga and Chi Kung, can help restore skin health and beauty by relieving pain, reducing inflammation, improving circulation, and activating regeneration and the removal of pigments and damaged proteins. Endorphins and encephalin are two peptides derived from the protein precursor pro-opiomelanocortin (POMC), and both can be produced by the brain and the skin. Another beneficial neurotransmitter is dopamine, which belongs to the catechol-

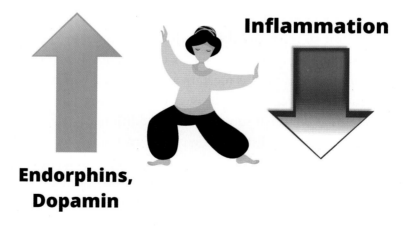

Figure 11.7. Chi Kung practices help increase "feel-good" molecules such as endorphins and dopamine, alleviating inflammation in the skin.

amine family and has been shown to produce the same beneficial effects in the skin as beta-endorphin. Dopamine is involved in feelings of motivation and pleasure, and its synthesis can be disrupted by molecules released during stress and with inflammation. Chi Kung, relaxation, meditation, and slow, mindful movements restore dopamine synthesis, bringing more pleasure and joy to life. This is one more reason why you should make relaxation the cornerstone of your beauty regimen.

ANGER, ANXIETY, AND ACNE

Acne is a chronic skin disorder that manifests as inflamed and enlarged sebaceous glands. It may be present at all times in various degrees of severity or come in flares, when relatively healthy and unaffected skin breaks out in pimples in response to emotional stress, alcohol, sugary food, and other influences. Acne is often considered an adolescent skin problem because 80 percent of people between thirteen and twenty-five have acne. However adult acne is no less a serious problem. Approximately 40 to 50 percent of people age twenty to thirty and 20 percent of those over forty have acne either constantly present or flaring up from time to time.

Even though acne is a dermatological problem, it has much wider implications. First, even mild acne negatively affects the skin's beauty. Second, acne can lead to psychological issues related to one's self-esteem and can get worse because of the stress these issues cause. Third, dermatological treatment of acne is often unsuccessful because it does not take into account one's emotions, skin-care regimen, and lifestyle. Just as with sun-induced skin damage, it is easier to understand acne when we focus on energy balance.

One of the manifestations of fire energy in the skin is inflammation, which has fire's burning, hot, flaring, flaming, and expanding qualities. An excess of fire energy in the skin can manifest as flushed skin, inflamed blood vessels, and puffiness in the face. Fire energy also is related to the negative emotional energies of hatred, rage, impatience, and judgment. These energies are fed by the wood energy of anger. At

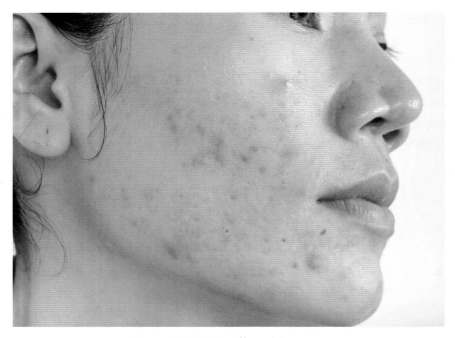

Figure 11.8. Skin affected by acne.

the same time, fear energy is related to the water element in the kidneys and can feed the wood energy of anger, which can feed the negative energies related to fire in the heart. Self-directed anger caused by self-judgment can generate anxiety and a physiological state of stress that leads to inflammation and skin damage. These conditions are all known to contribute to the worsening of adult acne.

A healthy sebaceous gland has an opening to the skin's surface—a pore—that releases skin oil. Some people have small sebaceous glands with barely visible pores, and other people have larger, more visible pores. The sebaceous gland's opening is covered by translucent, flat, hardened keratinous scales, which have to shed regularly to renew and regenerate. When skin oil is liquid and flows with ease, this process occurs without disrupting the skin's functioning. If, however, the skin oil becomes thicker, it can start forming a dense mix within the skin cells that clogs pore openings. Toxic irritants and inflammation, as well as excessive UV exposure, only increase the production of skin oil.

In young people, acne often appears in puberty because the male sexual hormone testosterone increases in both sexes during puberty and triggers elevated skin-oil production and enlargement of the sebaceous glands. By itself, testosterone does not increase skin oil, but it does so after it is converted into its active form, di-hydro-testosterone, or DHT, which stimulates skin-oil production. Acne may also increase in menopause due to the weakening of estrogen, which makes more testosterone available for converting into DHT.

Acne is also associated with a microorganism that is called *Propionibacterium acnes*. This microorganism inhabits sebaceous glands and feeds on skin oil, breaking it down into fatty acids. If the sebaceous glands function normally, this microorganism causes no harm. However if the sebaceous glands become blocked, enlarged, and produce more oil, this microorganism multiplies and starts causing the release of more fatty acids, which affects the normal development of skin cells and causes more irritation and inflammation. Once the pores become blocked and irritated, other microorganisms may start multiplying such as *Staphylococcus* and *Streptococcus* genuses. At this stage the person may need some serious dermatological help, which often involves the use of antibiotics and retinoids.

Acne is very much linked to stress and anger. In a 1988 study, dermatologists evaluated emotional and neurological associations in patients with various degrees of acne. It was found that anger and anxiety, but not other neurological or psychological states, are associated with the severity of acne. Researchers measured both "anger in," which is a self-directed anger, and "anger out," anger directed at others. Both were found to be associated with severe acne. This shows that not just anxiety but also various forms of anger contribute to the severity of acne.[10] Another study found that anger by itself does not significantly contribute to the severity of acne, but it does affect the overall quality of life and a person's adherence to a proper skin-care regimen and nutrition.[11]

One of the reasons science struggles to assess what role anger plays in acne is because psychological and self-reported evaluations of anger may be different from the actual effects of anger energy in the body.

One person may get angry quite often, but then release it just as quickly, with no ill effects. Another person may not even realize they're angry because they hold their anger in so tightly they only feel frustration, irritation, and self-judgment. Self-directed anger such as this is usually unconscious and manifests as persistent tension in the body—and, frequently, acne. The Tao believes that it is not the negative emotion itself but holding it in the body without release that causes issues.

When anger is held in the body, it fuels hatred, rage, judgment, impatience, and cruelty, which is directed at oneself and at others, which further increases skin damage and inflammation. This has been confirmed by another study in which it was demonstrated that it is not stress itself but a person's response to stress that affects acne severity. For example, people who use avoidance strategies in dealing with stress were shown to have a higher level of the inflammatory neuropeptide Substance P and, consequently, more severe acne.[12]

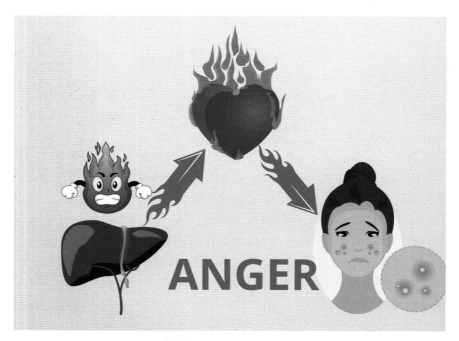

Figure 11.9. Anger in the liver creates excess fire energy in the heart, affecting the skin.

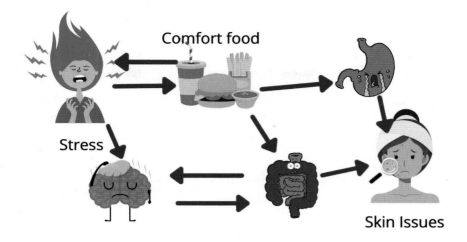

Figure 11.10. Unbalanced emotions, unbalanced nutrition, and unbalanced gut microflora create a vicious cycle of acne and inflammation in the skin.

Acne severity is also linked to the health of gut microflora. At the same time, gut microflora is affected by both emotional stress and unhealthy low-fiber food such as junk food and sugar, which people tend to eat in response to stress. Unbalanced gut microflora can release chemicals that increase anger and anxiety. Therefore unbalanced emotions, unbalanced nutrition, and unbalanced gut microflora create a vicious cycle, resulting in increased oil production, more inflammation, moodiness and depression, and, as a result, skin problems such as acne.

THE BRAIN-SKIN CONNECTION AND COSMETIC REMEDIES FOR ACNE

Many people who have oily, acne-prone skin use hot water, soap, and alcohol-based skin cleansers. They also get angry at their skin, depressed about their looks, and anxious and frustrated with remedies that don't work. All of this further aggravates acne. Many people will suntan excessively in the hopes of drying out their acne. However sun therapy works well only in moderation, while excessive exposure can further damage the skin. This is because there are many real links between the brain and the skin. One of them is through neuropeptides such as Substance P, which is released from nerve endings in the skin in response to irritation. Ironically, this chemical compound makes the skin oilier, increasing the production of skin oil and causing enlargement of the sebaceous glands. This makes evolutionary sense. In the past, if something continuously irritated an animal's skin, the reasonable response was to increase oil production to help protect the skin from the irritating substance. Today if we use irritating products to remove skin oil, the skin does not know this is the case—all it knows is that it's being exposed to an irritant, so it does its best to make more oil.

In humans, the nerves respond to our mental images as well as to external factors. The skin doesn't have its own eyes, so it has to trust what the brain communicates to it. And what the brain tells the skin is to release Substance P in response to emotional stress. Many people know that stress causes acne breakouts, but few truly understand the direct link to the brain, which is not only psychological but also chemical. In many cases, if you have acne, remaining in a stressed-out state is like putting more inflammatory chemicals into one's own skin. It is important to note that not all people who have acne have visibly oily

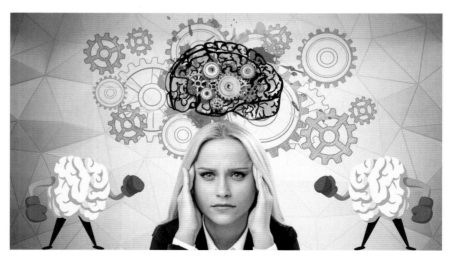

Figure 11.11. Stressful thoughts trigger a stress response in the skin.

skin. In many cases, the overall skin quality may be normal or even dry, while oil production in blocked oil glands may increase. In this case using harsh cleansers may cause even more skin dryness and sensitivity, as well as further irritation.

The Six Golden Rules of Skin Care for Acne-Prone Skin

1. **Be gentle:** It is important to use a very mild skin cleanser and avoid any product containing alcohol or other harsh solvents.
2. **Regularly exfoliate:** Use alpha-hydroxy acid-based products such as those containing glycolic or lactic acid to gently exfoliate your skin and open pores. Use salicylic acid-based products to reduce oiliness.
3. **Use probiotics for the skin and gut:** They will help balance your microflora.
4. **Avoid "oil-free" cosmetic products:** They often contain oil-like substances that do not feel oily but nevertheless can clog pores.
5. **Replenish skin antioxidants:** They help reduce free-radical damage in skin.
6. **Use skin-care products with natural antibacterial and anti-inflammatory extracts:** Such natural compounds as white willow bark extract, tea tree oil, natural clay, and Dead Sea salts can soothe the skin and reduce breakouts.

In addition to these measures, the biggest breakthrough will come from restoring the energy balance in the skin and body through Chi Kung practice. This means balancing fire energy and turning a conflict cycle back into a creating cycle.

ROSACEA AND SUN SENSITIVITY

Some people, especially those with pale, thin, easily blushing skin, are highly sensitive to cosmetics, cold, wind, alcohol, and spicy foods, and when exposed to these irritatants their skin becomes red and splotchy.

Outbreaks of small reddish bumps on the forehead and the nose as well as areas of flaky and dry skin are a sign of rosacea.

Rosacea currently affects around 5.5 percent of the adult population globally.[13] It mostly affects fair-skinned people of Northern European ancestry (Scandinavia, Germany, England, etc.); however, other skin types may be affected too. Rosacea may at first manifest only as a tendency to blush easily, a sensitivity to cosmetics, and a tendency for redness of the nose and cheeks after being out in the cold, eating spicy foods, or drinking alcohol. Over time, rosacea can resemble acne and cause skin flaking, a reddish rash, swelling, and even enlargement of the nose, which often gives the impression that the person is an alcoholic. Up until recently, many dermatologists called rosacea "adult acne" or "rosacea acne"; however, rosacea is completely unrelated to acne. In fact, many antiacne cosmetic products and over-the-counter medications may make rosacea worse by further disrupting the skin barrier, which is already compromised in rosacea. Any treatment for rosacea has to include hydration and restoration of barrier function.[14]

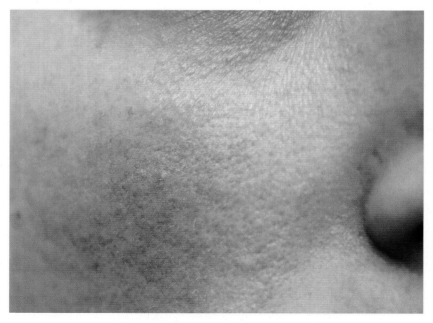

Figure 11.12. Close-up of skin with rosacea.

People who suffer from rosacea have a number of biological processes that are out of balance. First, they have an abnormally high production of antimicrobial peptides. This means their skin is always on high alert. People with rosacea also have a tendency to produce more free radicals of oxygen (ROS) in response to UV light, microbes, irritants, and other environmental threats. This means that skin affected by rosacea overreacts to stressors that would not affect healthy skin.[15] Therefore balancing of emotional energy for rocasea has to be focused more on balancing fear energy than anger energy. Fear is linked to the water element in the kidneys and can feed anger (wood energy) in the liver and fire energy in the heart, which in turn can feed anxiety and doubt in the spleen, bringing more power to the fear in the kidneys.

Five Golden Rules of Skin-Care for Rosacea

1. **Avoid irritants:** With rosacea, anything that activates the skin's defensive mechanisms can cause the abnormal production of antimicrobial peptides, the generation of ROS, and inflammation. Every time this happens, the condition progresses a step further. Wash your face with only neutral (around pH 7), very mild cleansers. Avoid harsh alkaline soaps, alcohol-based cleansers, and hot and very cold water. After washing your face, gently pat it with a soft towel and do not rub. If you wish you can apply a thin coat of protective moisturizer, but make sure it is suitable for very sensitive skin.

2. **Protect against excessive UV radiation:** It is advisable to expose the skin to sunlight in the morning hours for fifteen to thirty minutes. Whole-body exposure is best. At all other times use sun protection.

3. **Reduce inflammation:** Use gentle skin products containing natural soothing and anti-inflammatory ingredients. Some examples are witch hazel, chamomile, and lavender. Resveratrol, a compound found in red wine, is also useful to take as both a supplement and as an ingredient in skin-care products.

4. **Use gentle exfoliation:** Exfoliating clears flaky skin. Lactic acid is the mildest of alpha-hydroxy acids, and it is naturally present in the skin. It also has moisturizing properties.
5. **Use probiotics:** They balance the skin and gut microbiome.

RESTORING THE BALANCE OF THE FIVE ELEMENTS IN THE SKIN

As we read in chapter 4, Taoists long ago discovered that our emotions are related to the five natural elements, and they learned to balance them by applying their understanding of the qualities and powers of each element. For example, anger is related to the wood element and has a growing, expanding quality. When anger turns into rage, it is related to the fire element and has a hot, expanding, consuming quality. When anger is held in the body, it gives the skin a "wooden" quality that manifests as a hardened face, clenched jaws, and narrowed eyes. Greed and jealousy are also related to the wood element in the liver. When they are out of balance, people "turn green with envy." The person who is often angry, frustrated, and displeased is said to have a lot of bile. When anger turns into full, blazing, fiery rage, the skin turns red, the eyes start blazing with fire, the blood pressure may increase, and the heart beats faster. Fear, which is kidney/water energy, turns the skin pale and cold. Depression, sadness, and grief, which are connected to metal, make the skin look grayish and listless.

There are many psychological interventions for emotional imbalance, but the problem is that most of them are based on talk therapy, which relies on words to change emotional reactions, and this kind of process can take a very long time. Taoists discovered that they can work *directly* with patterns of emotional energy in the body to produce quick results. In balancing the five elements in the body we will still have negative emotions—after all, it's only human to have these feelings—but we can prevent them from affecting our health and the beauty of our skin.

To balance emotional energy, Taoists use the element of earth (spleen, stomach, and pancreas) as the balancing force. Planet Earth

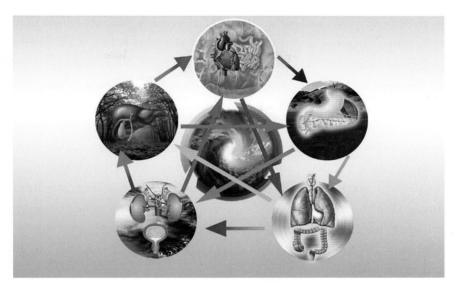

Figure 11.13. The emotions are related to the natural elements and can be balanced by understanding the qualities and powers of each element.

is very big and can attract and absorb negative energy. By learning to release our negative emotions down into the earth, we can remove any excess of elemental energy that is out of balance. The Tao says that unconditional love is the most powerful healing and balancing force there is. To use a gardening metaphor, love can be compared to a friendly microorganism that transforms all the garbage and food scraps we put in a compost pile into good, fertile nutrients for the soil that can be used to grow food and flowers.

In chapter 4 we examined how to balance the five elements through the Five Elements Creating Cycle, and in chapter 7 we discussed how to use the Six Healing Sounds to release negative energy at the end of the day. In chapter 10 we learned how to use a tree to help us quickly balance negative energy when one or more of the elements is noticeably out of balance and threatens to take over and disrupt the skin's flow. Trees are naturally connected to the earth and they can actually use our negative energy to nourish themselves. Because of their generous nature, trees are perfect for receiving the emotional energy related to the wood, water, and earth elements. By releasing doubts before they turn into depression and fear, and by releasing fear before it turns into anger and then rage, we can prevent the skin from overheating through an excess of fire energy. As you do these practices and meditations you should focus on those elements that are out of balance and spend more time releasing the excess of energy in those elements. In our world today, people often have an imbalance of fire and water, and we have considered the results of such an imbalance in various skin conditions. Since the heart works really hard, it is important not to let it overheat. So clearing the heart has to be a priority. The kidneys store the original life force energy, and having too much stress depletes this energy. Therefore the kidneys have to be regularly cleared of negative energy and replenished.

The following version of the Inner Smile focuses on the heart and kidneys as well as on replenishing one's unconditional love energy.

The Inner Smile for Balancing Excess Fire and Water Energy

1. Take a deep breath, smile, look into your heart, and become aware of the fire element in your heart. As you smile into your heart, spiral your eyes in your heart, gathering all the excess heat and burning energy. Exhale with the sound *haaawwwww*. The fire element is connected to the heart and small intestine. It is connected to the positive emotions of love, joy, and happiness, as well as to the negative emotions of hatred, cruelty, judgment, impatience, and rage. It is related to the south, to the color red, to the season of summer, to the planet Mars, and to a sacred animal, the red pheasant. An imbalance of fire in the skin is perceived as burning, hot, pressure, red spots, blisters, and swelling. Whether the imbalance is created by excessive exposure to the sun's ultraviolet rays, a hot environment, or burning emotions, the result is that it will increase inflammation, cause irritation, and accelerate aging. Use the sound *haaawwwww* to release excess heat from the heart.

2. Become aware of the water element and your kidneys. This is connected to the positive states of calmness, gentleness, and tranquility, and to the negative emotion of fear, which is often caused by trauma or shock. It is also connected to the north, the color blue, the season of winter, the planet Mercury, and a sacred animal, the blue turtle. An imbalance of water energy in the skin manifests as paleness, coldness, goosebumps, flakiness, lifelessness, and tension. To release excess water energy from the kidneys, use the sound *chooooooo*. Also, moving cooler, calming energy from your kidneys to your heart with the sound *chooooooo,* and moving heat from your heart to your kidneys with the sound *haaawwwww,* will balance your energy. You can spend a longer amount of time cooling down your heart because it very easily overheats and throws all the other elements out of balance. Remember to smile.

3. When you feel your heart is clean and clear and your kidneys are warm and calm, bring your awareness to your crown and third eye. Look through your third eye out into the universe. Then look into your heart and find the frequency of unconditional love there. Inhale the love in your heart and exhale that love out into the universe. Imagine that frequency of love being sent to galaxies far away. Become aware of the unconditional love that permeates the universe. Inhale unconditional love energy through your third eye into your heart. As you inhale universal unconditional love into your heart, feel it increasing. Keep smiling into your heart and let the love energy increase even more. Then inhale love from your heart and exhale it through your third eye back out into the universe. Inhale unconditional love from the universe and exhale it into your heart. Feel your heart being balanced by unconditional love.

4. Smile into your spleen and guide unconditional love from your heart into your spleen, pancreas, and stomach. Keep smiling into your spleen and feel it being balanced. Return to your heart.

5. Smile into your lungs and guide universal unconditional love from your heart into your lungs. Keep smiling into your lungs and feel them returning to balance. Return to your heart.

6. Smile into your kidneys and guide universal unconditional love from your heart into your kidneys. Feel your kidneys returning to balance. Return to your heart.

7. Smile into your liver and guide unconditional love from your heart into your liver. Feel your liver returning to balance. Return to your heart.

8. Keep going back to your heart and replenishing the unconditional love flowing to and from the universe. Go through all your organs nine times until they all are in balance.

9. Breathe and smile red light, love, joy, and happiness from your heart into your skin. Breathe and smile golden light, trust, confidence, and hope from your spleen, pancreas, and stomach into your skin. Breathe and smile white light, courage, and fairness from your lungs into your skin. Breathe and smile blue light, calmness, tranquility, and gentleness from your kidneys into your skin. Finally, breathe green light, kindness, and generosity from your liver into your skin. Smile all over yourself and let unconditional love from the universe flow through your skin from your crown and third eye and then down to the rest of your body, like a waterfall.

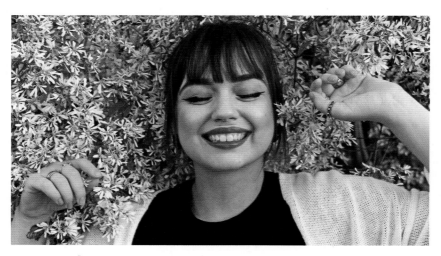

Figure 11.14. The Inner Smile—smiling down to all your organs to balance your skin.

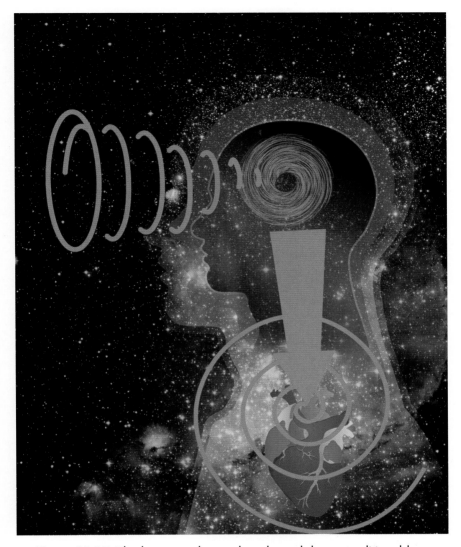

Figure 11.15. The heart can be used to channel the unconditional love
of the universe to your organs and skin, and then back again
to the universe.

Once your heart is clear of excess energy and no longer blocked or overheated, it can channel pure, unconditional love from the universe to help
balance all the other organs.

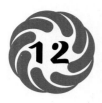

Five Elements Nutrition for Skin Beauty

The skin's vitality and beauty are closely connected to the health and vitality of the digestive system. Ancient Taoists placed great importance on digestion, absorption, and elimination, and believed that when these three key processes are taken care of, the whole body reflects a state of health. Today, many people try one diet after another in search of a panacea that will help them lose weight and become healthier and happier, and be the cure-all for all their problems. Unfortunately, many diets do not take into account the needs of the skin, and some diets can even accelerate aging by creating a deficiency of important nutritional elements or increasing inflammation.

The skin cannot feed itself and protect itself from the many harmful ingredients present in much of what passes for food. Therefore its health and beauty depend on our food choices. As the largest organ of the body, one that continuously repairs and renews itself, the skin stands between our inner universe and the universe around us, and it requires food with nourishing and protective nutrients to help it stay beautiful and radiant.

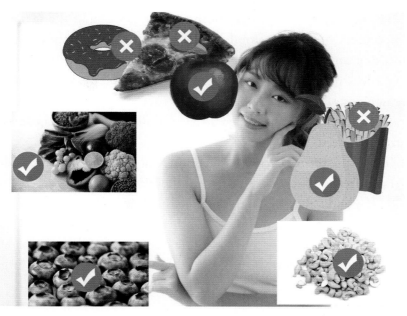

Figure 12.1. Food can repair, renew, and protect the skin, or it can damage it if we indulge in food with little nutritional value.

In 1989, Stephen DeFelice, M.D., founder and chairman of the Foundation for Innovation in Medicine, was the first to coin the term *nutraceutical,* a combination of *nutrition* and *pharmaceutical.* DeFelice defined nutraceuticals as "food (or a part of it) that provides medical or health benefits, including the prevention and/or treatment of a disease."[1]

Modern nutraceuticals may be used to improve health, delay the aging process, prevent chronic diseases such as obesity, increase life expectancy, and support the structure or functioning of the body. Certain foods can trigger or worsen pathological skin conditions such as acne, eczema, dermatitis, and others, and accelerate skin aging. At the same time, biologically active compounds in food can help the skin deal with environmental challenges, slow down aging, reduce inflammation, improve immunity and antioxidant defense, and boost overall health. Recent studies have confirmed that certain compounds in food, such as resveratrol from red wine or flavonoids from plants, can change the expression of various genes and rejuvenate our DNA.[2]

As modern science studies both the dangerous and the beneficial compounds in common food products, nutrition experts are giving confusing and conflicting information to a bewildered public. The weight-loss industry is big business. There is a plethora of books on any number of diets, while health food stores are filled with bottles of vitamins and herbal supplements that promise to meet every kind of nutritional need.

Taoist masters understand something very important that modern science often misses: food is the link between chi in nature and chi inside the body. Every living thing needs chi, including, of course, the human body. Chi can only flow when there is a balance of yin and yang. Taoists reasoned that the sun, a gigantic ball of blazing hot plasma with nuclear fusion reactions in its core, is the main source of hot, bright, expanding yang energy. Earth, in contrast, is dark, dense, and fertile with yin energy. Together, the yin and yang of Earth and the sun give

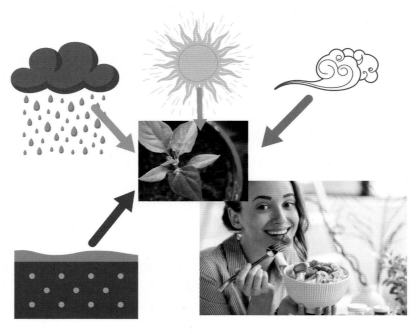

Figure 12.2. Food is the link between the elemental energy of nature and the human body.

birth to nature, including humanity itself. Earth is a living organism that feeds on the sun's energy, creating various life forms. Water flows through the body of Earth like the way chi, or electromagnetic energy, flows through the human body. Water and earth grow wood, like the way our body grows living cells when nourished with chi. Yin water warmed by fire evaporates and becomes yang steam. Similarly, electromagnetic yin energy in the human body, combined with the fire of consciousness, becomes the bright and expanding energy of the mind and spirit, and this energy shines through our skin and eyes, creating radiance and beauty.

All life forms on Earth have to tap into the abundant and omnipresent universal chi. There has to be a means by which living beings gather energy and process it, transforming it into the building blocks of life and physical energy. Plants, which evolved first on Earth, learned how to absorb solar radiation directly by using chlorophyl. Animals, which came next, learned to eat plants and other animals, too, to obtain chi. Animals need oxygen to burn the nutrients they eat in order to transform them into energy, or chi, so they breathe air and release CO_2, which in turn is used by plants. Plants reciprocate by releasing oxygen, which animals need. The air and water vapor in the atmosphere create a kind of planetary "skin" that protects Earth's body from dangerous cosmic radiation and helps preserve heat and moisture (fig. 12.3, p. 254). When viewed from this holistic perspective, the food that we consume becomes a precious gift of Earth, with our body being a part of Earth's energy flow. By learning how to make the most of the food we eat and use it to heal and nourish the body with love, we can make our skin healthier and more beautiful.

In the past, Taoist masters didn't have to deal with as many toxins in their food supply (with the exception of natural poisons in plants) as we do now. Yet even back when food was relatively clean and pure, they noticed that food can either poison or heal the body. Today, many foods in our diet are a curious mixture of pure, elemental, natural energy, along with a slew of artificial additives, many of which are quite new and foreign to the human body. The same food can be more or less nourishing

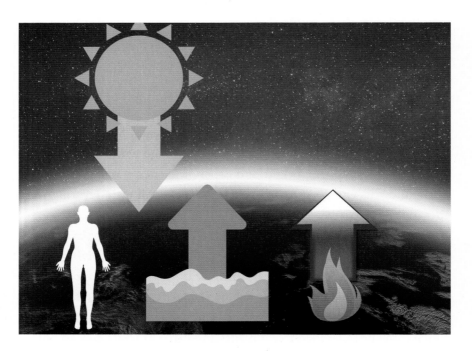

Figure 12.3. The atmosphere is like a skin that protects Earth's body from solar radiation and preserves moisture and heat.

depending on how it was grown and processed. It goes without saying that a vegetable picked right from the garden, grown in a toxin-free environment, minimally cooked or eaten raw, will supply the body with more vibrant elemental chi than a vegetable that was sprayed with pesticides, transported thousands of miles, processed with high heat and chemicals, mixed with artificial "enhancers," and stored for months or even years in a sealed plastic package.

The Nine Rules of Good Nutrition

1. **Eat colors in balance.** Eat foods that have a balanced ratio of five colors related to the five elements, which are red, yellow, white, blue, and green; this will ensure the balance of the five elements.

2. **If an organ is weak, eat more food with colors related to the organ's element.** For example, eating more green foods will make

your eyes, which are related to the wood element, the liver, and the color green, stronger and healthier.

3. **Eat food in season, and eat locally.** Foods that are stored for months or that are transported long distances have less chi compared to locally grown foods.

4. **Drink your food, chew your liquids.** Taoist masters have long proclaimed the benefits of slow, mindful eating. They advise us to chew food so well it becomes liquid. They even advise "chewing" liquids, by moving your teeth, to mix liquids with saliva and ensure best digestion.

5. **In the morning, eat like a king; during the day, eat like a prince; and in the evening, eat like a beggar.** Taoists believe we should not overload the digestive system before sleep. Modern science confirms that the body has its innate natural rhythms and it is best when food intake is aligned with these rhythms.[3]

6. **One third of what's on your plate feeds you, another third feeds the doctor, and the last third feeds the undertaker.** Eating in moderation is a prerequisite for good health.

7. **Avoid alcohol and stimulants.** Alcohol is basically a toxin, so the liver has to process and neutralize it, which wastes chi. Taoists believe that people who overconsume alcohol cannot control their energy and are more likely to waste it or let it be destructive. Stimulants such as coffee trick the body into releasing chi stored as a reserve. This further depletes chi and accelerates aging.

8. **Drink enough pure, clean water.** Our cells need water. Clean, pure water is best for dissolving and removing toxins and hydrating living tissues.

9. **Add additional good chi to your food.** Taoist masters recommended eating in a beautiful natural place or imagining a beautiful natural landscape while eating. Adding additional good chi to what we eat helps make the body and skin more beautiful and radiant.

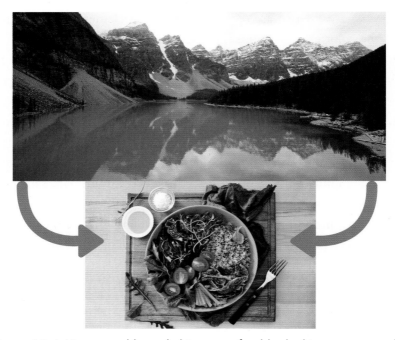

Figure 12.4. You can add good chi to your food by looking at nature while eating or imagining beautiful natural scenes when eating.

EATING VIBRANT COLORS

Including more colors in your food actually makes a lot of sense, because colorful, vibrant plants supply the human body with more than needed proteins, fats, and carbohydrates. It is now well-known that the same compounds that are responsible for plants' colors are also responsible for their protective, medicinal, and beautifying properties. Beneficial plant compounds are present in vibrantly colored vegetables, berries, fruits, spices, and medicinal herbs. Today many cosmetic companies offer "nutricosmetics," which are dietary supplements specifically designed to support the skin's health and beauty. Yet many people often forget that no pill can ever replace perfectly balanced natural elixirs created by Mother Nature, who is the best pharmacist and alchemist.

One of the reasons why plants are so good at creating protective and medicinal compounds is that a plant, unlike most animals, is attached to the ground. A plant cannot walk away from a pest or a plant-eating animal. A plant cannot escape the sun, wind, and freezing temperatures. A plant has to endure whatever conditions exist in its immediate environment or else it perishes. So plants produce a wide array of powerful biologically active compounds that allow them to adapt and survive. Since animals and plants evolved alongside each other for billions of years, animals learned to use the protective compounds from plants to protect and heal their own bodies. Many essential nutrients, such as vitamin C, are not produced in the human body and can be only be found in fruits and vegetables. Even though it is now convenient to buy a bottle of multivitamins, the truth is that it is much better for your body to consume food that contains those healthy vitamins in their natural, living form.

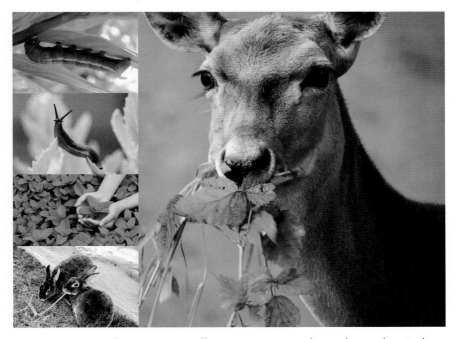

Figure 12.5. Plants cannot walk or run away, so they rely on chemical compounds to protect them. Animals receive many such protective compounds from eating these plants.

Of course, just because a chemical compound is found in plants does not automatically make it wholesome and beneficial. Some plant compounds are poisonous and best avoided. Since prehistory, humans have had to distinguish between food that can sustain and nourish the body and food that can damage it. This is why all animals, including humans, are equipped with a certain body sense that allows them to intuitively know which foods are best for them and which foods are best avoided. This system, endowed by nature, is not infallible, though. The modern food industry uses food additives to create enticing combinations of flavors to excite human taste buds and trick the body into not only accepting but craving food that is harmful to our health. Salt and sugar are two substances used to make food more addictive and to disable the body's inner radar. Many modern people, especially busy professionals who do not have time to cook as well as impoverished citizens who find fresh fruits and vegetables too expensive, eat meat almost exclusively, with a very limited selection of plant-based food. Oftentimes even if vegetables are included, they are cooked and processed beyond recognition and hence lack any useful biologically active compounds. Some examples are potato chips, popcorn, and boxed cereals said to contain dried fruit. Even though such foods are made to appear really attractive, they have a very limited amount, if any, of the kind of biologically active compounds essential for the body's health and the skin's beauty.

It is important to understand that even though many essential nutrients can be obtained from both animal and plant-based foods, plants contain a much wider selection of unique protective and beautifying compounds, many of which are not produced in the human body. Even though it may take a while for some people to learn to include more vibrant colors in their diet, it is an essential step. It is equally important to remember that enjoying delicious food is also essential, so the focus should be not on limiting or avoiding, but on adding and including nutrients that are needed to make the skin healthy and beautiful.

VITAMIN A

Vitamin A is one of the essential compounds that plays a key role in supporting the skin's healthy appearance. In animal bodies it exists as a fat-soluble compound called *retinol* and its derivates, the retinyl esters (palmitate, propionate, and acetate). The best animal sources of vitamin A are egg yolks, liver, cheese, butter, and fish. In plants, vitamin A exists in its pre-vitamin form as beta-carotene, which is a pigment that gives vegetables such as carrots their vibrant color.

Vitamin A is the master manager of the skin's biochemistry. Vitamin A and its derivatives influence all skin cells, including keratinocytes, fibroblasts, melanocytes, and immune cells. It stimulates the production of the skin's proteins and the growth of the skin's cells and their timely exfoliation; it increases the synthesis of collagen and glycosaminoglycans in the dermis, thereby supporting the skin's structure; it protects the skin against UV radiation; and it regulates skin oil production. Derivatives of vitamin A such as retinol are used in dermatology to control acne. Retin-A is a prescription retinoid approved by the FDA to treat premature skin aging. Severe deficiency of vitamin A is now rare, and a moderate deficiency can

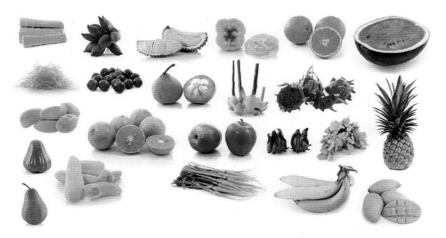

Figure 12.6. Examples of foods containing vitamin A and beta-carotene.

lead to accelerated skin aging and scaly, rough skin due to abnormal keratinization.

Both a deficiency and an excess of vitamin A is dangerous. Vitamin A significantly influences the skin's health and can be applied topically or taken in the form of food. It increases skin cell division when it is too slow, and slows it down if it is too fast. It reduces the skin's rate of exfoliation or accelerates it depending on the skin's needs. It improves hair growth and makes the skin appear younger and brighter. Retinoids can directly affect gene expression in the skin's cells, and they can increase or decrease the production of growth factors and other messengers. Vitamin A makes the epidermis more compact, thick, and firm. It also reduces the loss of water through the skin by fortifying the skin's barrier. Vitamin A improves the growth of new blood vessels in the dermis, restoring circulation and improving firmness and resilience of the dermis. Retinol esters in the skin's oil and stratum corneum can absorb ultraviolet light in the range of 300 to 350 nanometers, protecting the skin cells' DNA from damage. Since vitamin A regulates skin pigmentation, topically applied vitamin A in the form of retinoids can reduce pigment spots and other forms of sun-induced discoloration. Topical retinoids are also used to reduce wrinkles, increase firmness, and treat acne, rosacea, dermatitis, psoriasis, and cancerous growths.

In addition to beta-carotene, there are over a thousand different carotenoids in nature, many of which are present in food and have anti-oxidant and anti-inflammatory properties. They are the yellow, orange, and red pigments in pumpkins, sweet potatoes, sea buckthorn, salmon, shrimp, lobster, tomatoes, red and brown algae, and, of course, carrots. Studies have confirmed that a high carotenoid diet improves the skin's elasticity, smoothness, radiance, and beauty.[4]

Carotenoids play an important role in other organs, too. For example, lutein, meso-zeaxanthin, and zeaxanthin are important for our vision because they are pigments found in the macula of the eyes.[5]

VITAMIN C

Vitamin C, or L-ascorbic acid, is a vitamin compound derived from a sugar, D-glucose. Because the human body lacks the enzyme needed for the conversion of D-glucose into ascorbic acid, all our vitamin C needs have to be obtained from our food. The best sources are all the citrus fruits as well as black currants, strawberries, raspberries, kiwi fruit, cabbage (along with Brussels sprouts, broccoli, and cauliflower), spinach, red pepper, chives, parsley, hawthorn, and nettles. Some organs, such as the liver, pancreas, lungs, brain, and adrenal glands, can store vitamin C to help the body get through periods of deficiency.

In the past, sailors were terrified of a disease called scurvy, which would make their gums bleed and their teeth fall out, and in extreme cases would eventually lead to death. Scurvy is the consequence of an extreme vitamin C deficiency. Since there are no vegetables or fruits growing out at sea, long sea voyages would often put sailors at risk of developing scurvy. Today we know that vitamin C is a cofactor for an enzyme that catalyzes hydroxylation of the amino acids proline and lysine into hydroxyproline and hydroxylysine, which are used to build collagen. Vitamin C also activates the expression of collagen genes and stimulates skin fibroblasts, which are the cells responsible for collagen synthesis. The reason why scurvy was so deadly among seafarers in former times is because without vitamin C, the body cannot make collagen, which is a structural component for many tissues, including the skin.

The vitamin C concentration in the skin is 6–64 mg/100 grams net weight in the epidermis and 3–13 mg/100 grams in the dermis, which is higher than in other tissues. Vitamin C has a scientifically proven antiwrinkle effect, so many cosmetic companies now include it in their skin-care products. The main problem with vitamin C is that it is not stable in cosmetic products and can easily lose its activity, so manufacturers substitute a chemically modified form of vitamin C. But the best way to ensure that the skin has enough vitamin C is to simply eat more foods that contain it. Vitamin C is an important antioxidant that

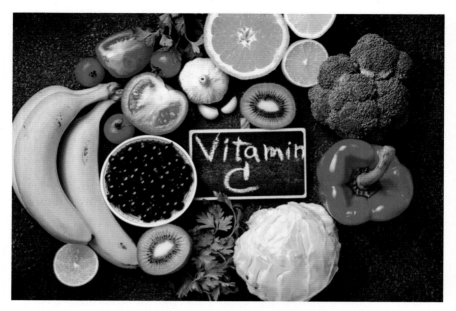

Figure 12.7. Examples of foods containing vitamin C.

together with vitamin E protects the skin from damage from the sun's ultraviolet radiation. It also controls the development of skin cells and the formation of the skin's barrier, as well as its hydration and production of glycosaminoglycans in the dermis.

Today, severe deficiency of vitamin C is rare, but since the skin is so dependent on vitamin C, even a moderate deficiency jeopardizes the skin's protection from the UV radiation, impairs its collagen synthesis, disrupts the skin's cell development, and weakens blood vessels, resulting in slow degeneration, easy bruising, delayed wound healing, and accelerated aging. Drinking orange and lemon juice and making sure we eat a wide range of colorful fruits and berries as well as dark green leafy vegetables will supply the skin with plenty of vitamin C.

VITAMIN E

Vitamin E, or tocopherol, is a fat-soluble vitamin found in vegetable oils such as wheat germ oil, sunflower oil, safflower oil, olive oil, coconut oil, and foods with a high oil content such as avocadoes and nuts (along with their oils). It is an essential antioxidant that plays a crucial role in the skin's defense against UV radiation and pollution. It participates in the biosynthesis of collagen, elastin, and glycosaminoglycans; reduces inflammation; and protects the skin's lipid barrier. Deficiencies of this vitamin are rare, since generally people have enough oil in their diet. However because vitamin E is easily depleted in its fight against free radicals, the skin can become deficient after prolonged exposure to UV radiation. With enough vitamin C, however, depleted vitamin E can be restored and regenerated, because in our cells these two anti-oxidants naturally work as a team restoring and regenerating each other as needed. Since vitamin C is water-soluble and found in the cyto-plasm of the cell while vitamin E is oil-soluble and found in the cellular membrane, nature designed a special mechanism that allows these two antioxidants to interact in the cellular membrane on the edge of the water-lipid line.

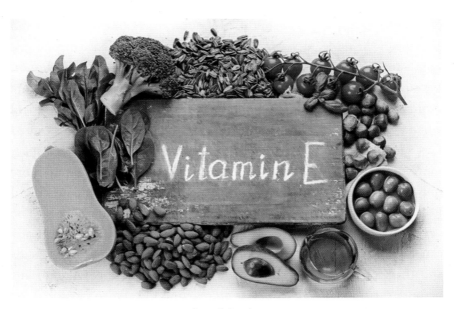

Figure 12.8. Examples of food containing vitamin E.

OMEGA 3 AND OMEGA 6

Many people who try to lose weight either avoid fats and oils or, depending on which diet they're following, do the opposite and try to avoid carbs and instead eat food containing vegetable fats and saturated animal fats. However those who are concerned with their skin's health and beauty need to know that the skin has special dietary needs when it comes to oils and fats, specifically omega 3 and omega 6 fats. Many common skin problems such as psoriasis, eczema, acne, dermatitis, rosacea, and dry skin can be helped by adjusting the ratio of these dietary oils, as a deficiency of omega 3 or omega 6 fats results in slack, wrinkled skin, increased sensitivity, and inflammation.

The body cannot function without lipids, which are fatty or waxy substances made by the body that don't dissolve in water and help with many of the body's functions. Dietary fats supply the basic building blocks of all lipid-based structures in the body such as cholesterol and fatty acids. There are two kinds of fatty acids, saturated and unsaturated. Unsaturated fatty acids are further divided to polyunsaturated and monounsaturated acids. The term *saturated* refers to the absence of double bonds in the chemical structure, which allows a more solid packing of the molecules. Monounsaturated fatty acids have one double bond, and polyunsaturated fatty acids have two or more double bonds. Because they do not have vulnerable double bonds, saturated fats are more resistant to oxidation, while polyunsaturated fats can go rancid when exposed to the air. Because of this structural difference, saturated fats, such as animal fats, which contain more saturated fatty acids, are more solid at room temperature. Unsaturated fats, which contain more polyunsaturated fats, remain liquid at room temperature and are found in vegetable oils. We need both kinds of fats, but we don't have to be overconcerned with having enough saturated fats because the body can make saturated fatty acids from carbohydrates and amino acids and therefore will never run out of saturated fats. This is important because the human body converts excess food into fat to be stored for leaner days when such foods may not be available. It cannot, however, manufacture certain unsaturated fatty acids—the essential polyunsaturated fatty acids (also called essential fats), such as what are found in vegetable oils, salmon, and nuts and seeds. These fatty acids, such as omega 6 and omega 3 fatty acids, are irreplaceable components of cellular membranes.

Cellular membranes are a special form of "skin" made of lipids that define and protect living cells. Just as we would not do well without our skin, we would not have a physical body without cellular membranes, as there would be no living cells. Cellular membranes are built from molecules called *phospholipids,* which have hydrophilic (meaning "attracted to water") "heads" comprised of a phosphorous residue, and two hydrophobic (meaning "afraid of water") "tails" comprised of fatty acids, which can be saturated, monounsaturated, or polyunsaturated. In a watery environment, hydrophobic tails try to get away from water, while hydrophilic heads want to interact with water. This allows phospholipids to form lipid bilayers, which are the basic structure of all

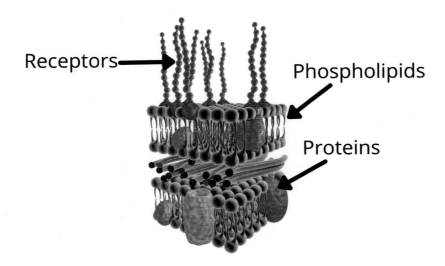

Figure 12.9. Biological membranes are made from phospholipids.

cellular membranes. Like the way skin serves as the boundary for the inner environment of the body and is equipped with sensory organs to receive signals from the outer environment, our cellular membranes serve as boundaries for our cells and are equipped with chemical sensors or receptors that receive signals from intercellular spaces.

Cellular membranes are important not only because they protect and define every living cell, but also because they transmit electromagnetic energy. Every cellular membrane is thus a medium for energy flow. Depending on what fatty acids are present in phospholipids, cellular membranes can be more liquid, or they can harden and become more solid, which affects their conductivity and flow. Too much saturated fat can makes cellular membranes hard and impedes energy flow, and for that reason consuming too much animal fat without balancing it with more liquid vegetable oils may affect the skin's health. On the other hand, cellular membranes do need some saturated fat and cholesterol to support their structure. Once again, as the Tao teaches, balance is key.

Another reason why balancing dietary fats is so important is because the fatty acids in our cellular membranes serve as a built-in emergency alert. Any break in a cellular membrane activates a special enzyme that starts cutting off fatty acid tails from phospholipids. At this point, other enzymes transform free fatty acids into immune-reactive molecules such as prostaglandins, eicosanoids, and others, which regulate inflammation, repair, and regeneration. Some polyunsaturated fatty acids such as the omega 3s (a designation based on their chemical structure) reduce inflammation, while others, the omega 6s, tend to increase inflammation. This supports the idea that food can be used to support one's health and vitality and can alleviate some common skin problems.

It would be so simple to say we should just avoid omega 6 fats, which are found in most common vegetable oils such as canola, corn, and sunflower, and instead consume more omega 3 oils such as flaxseed and fish. But omega 6 oils play a very special role in the skin. As discussed earlier, the skin has its own membrane structure, called the *epidermal barrier,* comprised of ceramides and sphingolipids. These molecules are also membrane-forming lipids that are both hydrophilic and hydrophobic. Their hydrophilic "head" is composed of sphingosine alcohol, while their lipophilic "tail" is a long-chained polyunsaturated fatty acid. Ceramides found in skin contain omega 6 fatty acids such as linoleic and gamma linoleic acid, which ensure integrity of the epidermal barrier.

Over the years, a great many studies have confirmed that to ensure skin integrity and health, omega 6 and omega 3 fatty acids have to be present in a *balanced* ratio. There are still discussions on what this perfect ratio should be, but most scientists agree that the omega 6 to omega 3 ratio should be should be between 2:1 and 4:1. The problem is that a typical Western diet has an omega 6:omega 3 ratio of 15:1, and therefore, contains too much omega 6 fat.[6]

People who have inflammatory skin conditions may need dietary supplements and topical application of plant oils that are rich in all required fatty acids together with liposoluble vitamins and other biologically active compounds. Among these are evening primrose, borage, wheat germ, avocado, grape seed, olive, black currant, and flax seed oil. For example, borage oil is rich in omega 6 gamma-linoleic fatty acid, or GLA, which is an omega 6 fatty acid that does not increase inflammation and helps improve skin barrier function,[7] while avocado oil, in addition to monosaturated and polyunsaturated fatty acids, is also rich in carotenoids, which have antioxidant and anti-inflammatory properties.[8] These oils reduce inflammation, redness, itching, and abnormal exfoliation of the skin. They are also very beneficial for the body in general, especially for brain health.[9]

Dietary oils also contain certain chemical compounds that are present in small amounts, but are very beneficial for the skin. These are beta-carotene, beta-sitosterol, vitamin E, squalene, and others. These compounds are known to reduce inflammation, slow down aging, increase regeneration, and have other positive effects. Oils rich in these health and beauty compounds are wheat germ, avocado, olive, and walnut oils. Good sources of omega 3 oils are fish oil and flaxseed oil. For a balanced omega 3 to omega 6 ratio, use dietary supplements containing borage, black currant, and evening primrose oils. Eating salmon, nuts, and avocados, and using cold-pressed vegetable oils raw (such as in salads) will help the skin receive necessary essential polyunsaturated fatty acids.

It's important that we avoid all hydrogenated oils or trans fats, which contain chemically modified fatty acids that disrupt the fine workings of cellular membranes and can increase inflammation and disrupt energy flow. When vegetable oils are used for high-temperature cooking they lose their beneficial qualities and may become harmful for skin.

PLANT POLYPHENOLS

Polyphenols are biologically active plant compounds found in fruits, vegetables, nuts, seeds, flowers, and bark. Polyphenols have strong antioxidant and anti-inflammatory activity and play an important role in protecting the skin from the damaging effects of UV radiation by preventing premature aging caused by it. Some of the most powerful polyphenols are the proanthocyanidins, which are found in grapes, red wine, and pine bark; the procyanidins, found in apples, grapes, cranberry, and pine bark; resveratrol (aka stilbene), found in red wine; phenolic acid, found in coffee and pomegranates; flavonoids, found in berries and fruits; catechins, found in green tea; and isoflavones, found in soy and other members of the bean family. Studies have demonstrated that polyphenols neutralize a wide range of reactive free radicals of oxygen, protecting the skin from oxidative damage, alleviating inflammation, supporting the immune system, stimulating DNA repair and skin renewal, and inhibiting development of some skin cancers.[10] All these benefits can be obtained by simply eating more colorful fruits and berries, as well as drinking green tea. The champions of the polyphenol world are grapes, apples, blueberries, acai berries, soy, green tea, and red wine.

AMINO ACIDS AND BIOLOGICAL PEPTIDES

Amino acids are best known as the building blocks of proteins, but they can also be metabolized into biologically active signal molecules such as hormones and neurotransmitters. For example, the amino acid tryptophan is a precursor of the neurotransmitter serotonin (which is responsible for feelings of happiness and joy), the hormone melatonin (a very important regulator of mood and sleep), and vitamin B_3 or niacinamide (which boosts cellular energy and has anti-inflammatory effects on skin). Tryptophan belongs to a family of essential amino acids that are not produced in the human body. Tyrosine is another essential amino acid that is metabolized in melanin, the skin's pigment.

In addition to amino acids, another group of important nutrients are the biologically active peptides, which are short-chain amino acids ranging from two or three to dozens of amino acids. One of the most studied biologically active peptides is the copper peptide GHK-Cu (glycyl-l-histidyl-l-lysine). This is a small molecule containing only three amino acids that has a high affinity to copper ions. GHK-Cu naturally occurs in the human body and is a part of the collagen molecule and some other structural proteins. GHK-Cu is a natural stimulator of skin regeneration, which can help switch the wound-healing process from inflammation to regeneration and healing.[11] Usually a well-balanced diet containing various food sources that can include animal products or be exclusively plant-based will supply the skin with essential amino acids. Collagen supplementation, however, can further improve skin texture, smoothness, and overall radiance.

MINERALS

A healthy diet should supply the skin with minerals such as calcium, phosphorus, potassium, sodium, and magnesium, as well as microelements such as selenium, zinc, iodine, sulphur, iron, cobalt, copper, manganese, and molybdenum. Many minerals, like vitamins, perform an important role as cofactors for enzymes. For example, copper, zinc, and magnesium are cofactors for the essential antioxidant enzyme super oxide dismutase (SOD), which protects the skin from oxidative damage and premature aging.

Selenium is a cofactor for the antioxidant enzyme glutathione peroxidase, which neutralizes hydrogen peroxide, one of the damaging oxidative chemicals produced when skin is exposed to UV radiation or has inflammation. Selenium is an important antiaging mineral that protects the skin from wrinkles caused specifically by UVA radiation. Selenium can be obtained from fish, eggs, mushrooms, spinach, lentils, bananas, cashew and brazil nuts, milk, and yogurt.

Zinc is a cofactor for over three hundred enzymes, and the skin is the third-ranking organ with the highest content of zinc. Zinc regulates immune functions, protein synthesis, and cell division, and improves survival of the skin cells and many other functions. Topical applications of zinc have been shown to improve skin regeneration and wound healing, slow down skin aging, reduce skin oiliness, and help treat many inflammatory skin conditions such as acne, rosacea, and eczema.[12] The best sources of zinc are meat, shellfish, legumes, hemp and squash seeds, nuts, eggs, and some whole grains such as buckwheat and quinoa.

Copper is another mineral that greatly affects the skin's health and beauty. It is an essential part of over thirty proteins required for proper functioning of the human body. Among them is lysyl oxidase, which is involved in collagen synthesis, and tyrosinase, an enzyme involved in the synthesis of the skin's pigment melanin. Copper regulates the growth and proliferation of skin cells and the activity of enzymes that break down the dermal matrix. It also stimulates the activity of fibroblasts, the cells that produce collagen, and regulates enzymes involved in DNA repair. Copper-containing peptides such as GHK-Cu are commonly used in the beauty industry, in antiaging and protective skin-care products. Rich sources of copper are organ meats (especially liver), shellfish, marine algae, legumes, nuts, and mushrooms.

After oxygen, silicon is the second most abundant element on earth, from which the chemical compound silica is derived. Dietary deficiency of silica is rare, however its availability decreases in tissues as we age because its absorption is regulated by the thymus gland, which atrophies with age. Silica is important for collagen and elastin synthesis, skin repair, and regeneration. As well, silica supplements are available for supporting the skin's health and beauty.

PROBIOTICS

The gut and the skin are allies. They talk to each other through signals sent through nerve fibers and chemical messengers. Therefore when there is inflammation and constipation in the intestines, the skin is always affected, and the results can be acne or psoriasis. To ensure that the intestines are healthy it is very important to add probiotics and fiber to one's diet.[13]

Beneficial gut microorganisms such as *Lactobacillus* and *Bifidobacterium* species produce a range of biologically active compounds that regulate mood, inflammation, and immune function. Even more important are healthy eating habits like mindful eating and sufficient chewing. Eating too fast, eating while distracted, and eating on the go contribute to bloating, indigestion, and constipation. Eating while stressed affects the gut's nervous system, our second brain, creating disturbances in the digestion. Minding the gut-skin-brain connection is a prerequisite to healthy and radiant skin.

THE EASY WAY TO EAT MINDFULLY

This chapter presents only some of the most essential nutrients that affect the skin. It is just as important to avoid toxins, including products treated with pesticides and other industrial toxins, alcohol, and food additives. Overly processed food provides very little life force. Too much sugar leads to accelerated aging of the skin's collagen and the formation of age spots due to a process called *protein glycation,* which is the chemical reaction of sugars with proteins that fuses proteins together; this process is the very one that creates a nice brown crust on grilled or deep-fried meat.

It may seem that you have to be a nutritionist or a chemist to under-stand all the dietary requirements and rules! Studying food chemistry and its relationship to the body can be exciting and fulfilling; however, for those who feel a bit overwhelmed with all this information, a much easier solution is to just follow the nine rules of good nutrition out-lined earlier in this chapter. When we eat fresh, local, and in season, and include all five vibrant colors, we will receive a plethora of benefi-cial biologically active compounds that will increase the skin's resilience, elasticity, and radiance. Plus, eating wholesome and vibrant food con-taining all five colors, with the full intention to savor and appreciate it, can be really enjoyable.

Foods That Supply Colors

- **Red and orange:** This includes red meat, salmon, shrimp, and red and orange vegetables, berries, and fruits. Eat carrots, pumpkin, sweet potatoes, tomatoes, winter squash, and red peppers. Fruits and berries include apples, blood oranges, red grapefruit, red grapes, strawberries, raspberries, red currants, goji berries, and papaya. It is believed that consuming more red and orange vegetables and fruits can help balance blood pressure, support the heart and blood vessels, and even reduce the risk of cancer. These colors can help protect the skin from UV-induced damage and pollutants, improve smoothness and elasticity, add vibrancy and radiance, and stimulate collagen and elastin.
- **Yellow:** These are egg yolks, cheese, butter, pineapple, bananas, yellow peppers, yellow squash, potatoes, honey, lemon, corn, turmeric, mango, jackfruit, and yellow plums. Like the red and orange foods, yellow food is rich in carotenoids. Bananas and cheese are also rich in the amino acid tryptophan, which makes serotonin, and potassium, which helps regulate blood pressure. Vegetable oils supply omega 3 and 6 fatty acids and are also con-sidered yellow food.

- **White:** These are egg whites, white meat, white fish, garlic, coconuts, onions, mushrooms, white beans, yogurt, and nuts such as cashews, sesame seeds, pine nuts, and peanuts. Many white foods are rich in potassium, fiber, beta-glucans, and lignans. White foods such as garlic, onions, and mushrooms support immunity and digestive health.

- **Blue:** These are plums, concord grapes, eggplant, blue tomatoes, purple potatoes, purple yam, purple asparagus, blue corn, blue potato, blue cheese, blue pea flower, and water. Blueberries especially are considered a superfood; they are rich in health-promoting nutrients such as plant polyphenols, vitamin C, carotenoids, and minerals.

- **Green:** These are all the leafy green vegetables (kale, chard, spinach, etc.), cucumbers, zucchini, broccoli, green apples, green grapes, asparagus, green cabbage, okra, celery, limes, peas, green beans, edamame, olives, and green tea. Green foods are full of essential vitamins, minerals, fiber, and vitamin C. Avocado especially is considered a superfood due to its rich content of vitamin E, dietary fiber, omega 6 oils, and the carotenoid lutein, which protects the eyes from age-related macular degeneration. Avocado is very high in lutein, 369 micrograms per fruit.

Food is the link between the five elements in nature and the five elements in our body. While it can be difficult to follow all the (often conflicting) dietary recommendations and watch all the nutrients we consume, it is much simpler and easier to be mindful of the five elements and their energy. Taoists say that eating food of certain colors helps add more chi to the corresponding organs: red and orange is for the fire element, which is the heart, small intestine, and tongue; yellow is for the earth element, which is the spleen, pancreas, and stomach, as well as the mouth; white is for the metal element, which is the lungs, large intestines, skin, immune system, and nose; blue is for the water element, which are the kidneys and ears; green is for the wood element, which is the liver and the eyes.

Mindful Chi Eating Principles

When we shift from eating unconsciously to mindful chi eating, it becomes clear that ensuring that our food contains good chi is no less important—and even more important—than counting calories, reading food labels, or watching the ratio of fats and carbs. Chi is real, and the food that enters our body will travel through the digestive tract and feed every cell. So it only makes sense to ensure that only good and vibrant chi enters our body when we eat.

- Make sure you set aside a quiet time for eating. It is best to ask your family to eat in silence for at least the first ten minutes, and only afterward engage in conversation. If this is impossible, limit the topics of conversation to those that bring good chi to the table.
- Put away all electronic devices and other distractions while eating. Food is a gift of the earth, and it is important to appreciate it.

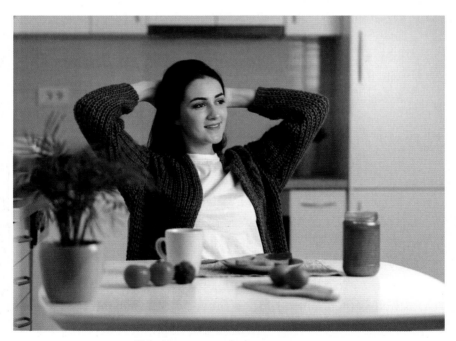

Figure 12.10. Mindful chi eating includes arranging your space, putting away electronics and distractions, and sending good chi into your meal.

- Clear your dining table from clutter and arrange it with love. You can look at a photograph of a beautiful place or recall a beautiful place in nature that you know. Imagine inhaling beautiful chi and mixing it into your food as you eat. You will notice that you will be more satisfied with less food, and your body will feel lighter and more uplifted.

- Before you start eating, take a moment to look at your plate and notice the colors. Use your eyes to welcome food into your body. Feel what kind of energy this food emanates. Appreciate this energy. Smell the aroma of your food.

- Smile into your food. Imagine directing good energy toward your food and mixing it in. In many cultures there is the custom of saying a prayer or blessing before eating a meal. This is because food, just like anything material, can absorb chi, including the chi of our thoughts.

- Take time to chew your food at least forty or fifty times. By doing this you will notice better digestion and more satisfaction from less food. Focus on the sensations in your mouth, on your tongue, and in your throat and belly as you chew. Smile into your body.

- It is important to stop eating when there is still room in your stomach. The stomach needs to move in order to digest food. When the stomach is overstretched with too much food, that food may pass down into the intestines before it is properly processed by the stomach, which will create distension, congestion, and gas in the intestines. Slow, mindful eating allows you to notice when you've had enough.

- When you're done eating, smile all over yourself and send gratitude to nature, the earth, the sun, and all the people who made it possible for you to eat the food you've just consumed.

- If you happened to eat too fast or you've eaten food that is not very wholesome, forgive yourself. Smile into your own heart. The more you forgive yourself and appreciate every little step, the more you will enjoy mindful chi eating.

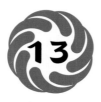

Chi Kung for Beautiful Hair

Ancient Taoist masters held that every hair extends from the skin like an antenna that can receive and transmit chi. They therefore placed great importance on hair vitality and strength. Longer and healthier hair allows for a better transmission of chi, while short, dry, brittle hair may not transmit as well.

Hair is one of the most noticeable characteristics of sexual attraction, beauty, confidence, and self-worth. Hair reflects social status, personal beliefs, and the state of one's health and hygiene. Thick, lustrous, healthy hair attracts attention and frames the face, defining and completing it. Hair loss can cause considerable emotional distress in both sexes, but is usually more devastating for women due to social conditioning, which attaches greater importance to hair as an aspect of a woman's beauty. Today hair health is plagued by a host of environmental and internal problems. Pollutants in the air, earth, water, and food; chemicals in the skin and in hair products; frequent washing with hot water and shampoos; tight hair bands; drying with hot air; hair dyes, permanent curling, and straightening; UV radiation and hormonal changes in menopause—all these affect hair vitality and beauty, causing premature graying, thinning, hair loss, itchy scalp, dandruff, and brittle ends. In this chapter we review the basics of hair physiology and discuss the Taoist approach to restoring beautiful hair.

HAIR IS PART OF THE SKIN

Even though hair appears to be different from skin, it is an integral part of it and is affected by the very same factors. Ironically, many methods that claim to make hair healthier and more beautiful in reality contribute to hair thinning and hair loss.

Seven Things to Know about Hair

1. **Hair is a mirror of the body.** Like the skin, hair reflects the state of a person's health and vitality and is affected by nutrition, internal problems, and emotions.

2. **Some hair loss is normal.** Hair growth is cyclic and includes phases of growth, regression of the hair follicle, and rest (explained below).

3. **Male and female sex hormones affect hair.** Biologically, hair growth pattern is different for men and for women. This means that hair responds to male and female sex hormones differently, depending on where it's growing. Hair on the face is stimulated by male sex hormones and suppressed by female sex hormones. Hair on the head is stimulated by female sex hormones and may be suppressed by male sex hormones.

4. **Hair is a sponge for chemicals.** Hair absorbs heavy metals, drugs, and other chemicals, depositing them in its structure.

5. **Hair cannot be repaired.** Only hair follicles can be regenerated, while hair itself is not a living structure.

6. **What damages the skin damages hair.** Hot water, detergents, toxic chemicals, ultraviolet radiation, poor nutrition, lack of adequate blood flow, pollution, dryness, stress, and hormonal imbalance all affect hair growth and beauty.

7. **Beautiful hair is a better antenna.** Dry, dead, brittle hair cannot receive and transmit chi.

The best way to understand hair is to think of it as being like a tree growing from deep in the earth. Like a tree, hair has roots—the hair

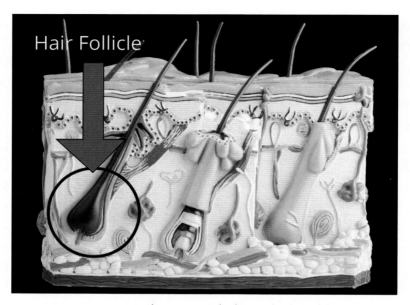

Figure 13.1. Hair has roots, which are the hair follicles.

follicles. Hair follicles contain stem cells that produce six rings of growing cells. The three inner rings create the medulla, which is the softer and more fragile part of the hair, and the three outer rings produce the hair cortex and cuticle.

The cuticle of hair consists of several layers of flattened, keratinized cells that wrap around the cortex. They are very similar to the keratinized cells of the skin's stratum corneum, and resemble scales. They serve the same functions as on the skin, providing strength, flexibility, protection, and waterproofing. Also like the skin, hair is protected by lipids that prevent water from getting inside the hair shaft, making hair flexible and smooth. Only instead of ceramides, hair is protected by omega 3 fatty acids, which are linked to keratin proteins.

The medulla does not contain living cells and is built from keratin fibers. Every keratin strand has repeating segments of the keratin molecule, a long protein molecule made of amino acids. Both the cortex and the medulla are made of keratin, but the medulla is spongier and can deliver moisture to the hair. The cortex is another structure made of keratinous fibrils produced by cells growing within the hair follicle. The keratinous fibrils that make up the cortex are sturdy and strong and are woven together like many wires inside a high-voltage electrical cable.

Only the very base of hair, where it meets the scalp, is alive, which means it contains living cells while the rest of hair does not. Because hair is not a living structure, it can be cut, colored, curled, straightened, and covered in various chemical substances. However it also means that once hair has emerged from the hair follicle, it cannot be repaired and regenerated other than through improving the skin or hair follicles. The rest of the hair can be cleaned, lubricated, softened, curled, dyed, or perfumed, but not really repaired. This is why the hair that frames our face looks more alive compared to hair ends, which are drier and more brittle. The only way to deal with dry and brittle hair is to cut it off and grow new hair.

THE HAIR GROWTH CYCLE

At any point in time there is hair that is actively growing, hair that is no longer growing, and hair that is ready to fall out. The cycle of growth of hair includes the growing phase, or anagen (2–8 years); the regression phase, or catagen (4–6 weeks); and the resting phase, or telogen (2–3 months).

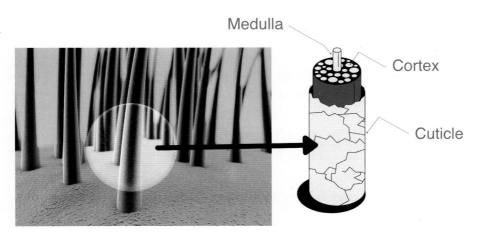

Figure 13.2. Structure of hair.

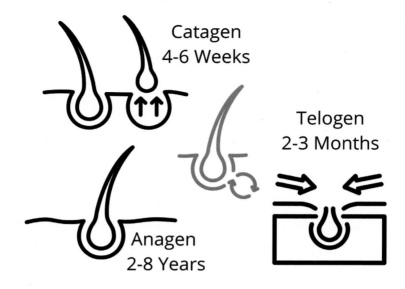

Figure 13.3. The hair growth cycle.

Usually around 90 to 95 percent of the hair on the head is in the anagen phase. During this growth phase, the follicular cells have to work really hard, making the proteins, lipids, and pigments required to create hair. Next, the cells deplete their resources and enter a regression stage during which the follicle shrinks and the hair is no longer growing. Finally, the follicle stops shrinking and just sits in the skin resting. At the end of telogen, the old hair falls out (usually during combing or washing), and the follicle starts growing new hair.

At first, a growing hair follicle produces a short, fine vellus hair, the hair that is found on most surfaces of the body in which the hair shaft lacks the central inner layer found in mature hair. It then matures into thick terminal hair. Since humans do not have fur covering their bodies, most of their skin produces thin, lightly pigmented, barely noticeable vellus hair with the exception of armpit hair and pubic hair, which becomes terminal hair after puberty. Men also have terminal facial hair such as that found in a beard or mustache. Women typically have less hair on their body and face compared to men, and most of this hair is soft and very thin vellus hair.

The growth cycle determines how much hair we have on our head and how long we can grow it. The longer the growing phase, the longer the hair. The shorter the resting phase, the more hair we have. An average length of anagen for most modern people is two to three years, and this allows us to grow hair only down to shoulder length at most. Those who have a longer anagen phase, five or more years, can grow hair waist-length. A healthy person loses about 100 to 150 hairs every day, which are replaced by approximately the same amount of growing hair. If the hair follicles take too long to replenish, then hair loss may start exceeding hair growth, and the hair will become thinner.

Robust, healthy, vigorous hair follicles produce thick, shiny, beautiful hair. Smaller, weaker, sickly hair follicles produce thinner and weaker hair. Since hair growth requires follicle cells to constantly produce more proteins and melanin, hair follicles require good circulation, swift removal of toxins, and a lot of energy. So the length, thickness, density, and health of hair, as well as its pigmentation, depends on hair follicle energy flow, which depends on the skin's energy flow. The hair growth cycle also is affected by age, ethnicity, and genetics.

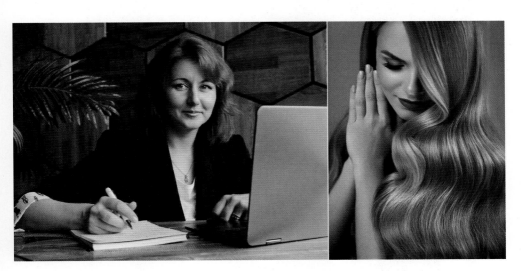

Figure 13.4. Hair follicles that remain in the growing phase for two to three years can grow only shoulder-length hair, while hair follicles that can grow for five or more years can grow waist-length hair.
Photo on the left by Gveter2.

HAIR AS A KEY INDICATOR

Hair is an important indicator of a person's vitality and vigor. A young, healthy, vital body usually features healthy, shiny, thick hair. Hair is a key component of personal identity. For women probably more so than men, hair is an essential component of one's personal beauty and identity. For both sexes, one's personal appearance differs significantly depending on hair color, style, length, thickness, vitality, and cleanliness. In many cultures, hairstyle and hair accessories are important indicators of social status. Changes in hairstyling and hair dress traditionally indicate changes in life such as maturity, marriage, mourning, going to war, and changes in social status. Monks and nuns shaved their heads to indicate relinquishing the physical desires and vanity of the mundane world. In the military, a close-cut, uniform haircut serves both hygienic and unifying purposes. In many cultures, married women cover their hair, allowing only their

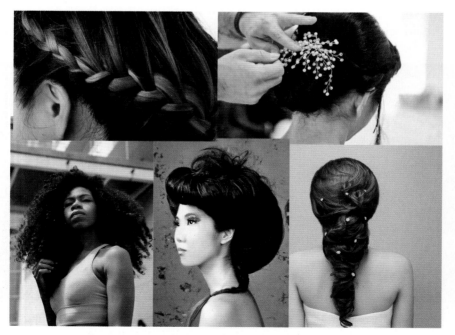

Figure 13.5. Hair can be styled and decorated to express individuality or to indicate one's cultural or social status.

husbands to see it. Not only Taoists, but many other indigenous cultures have cherished long, healthy hair. For example, Native Americans wore their hair long because they believed it connected them to the earth and nature and helped preserve mental and physical strength. That is why cutting or shaving a person's hair was a tactic used by colonizers to humiliate the colonized or the imprisoned to take away their power.

We may agree or disagree with placing importance on such a feature as hair, but biologically there is a reason why humans cannot help but respond to hair beauty and vitality. In prehistoric times, early humans had to be able to make very fast, split-second judgments about another human being, who could be either a friend, a foe, or a potential mate. Because hair can be seen from far away, those humans who became very good at noticing it survived and left offspring. So the habit of quickly noticing hair and making swift decisions based on it became embedded in our neurology and is therefore very hard to change. Hair length, thickness, and hairstyle play a major role in physical attraction between the sexes. Therefore such problems as hair loss, thinning, graying, and loss of hair vitality may cause significant emotional distress and affect people's sense of self-worth and beauty.

Ten Factors That Influence Hair Vitality and Growth

1. **Age:** As skin and body regeneration slows down, the hair becomes thinner, drier, less pigmented, and eventually turns gray. Men may grow bald, and women may start losing hair.

2. **Sex hormones:** Sex hormones stimulate hair growth in the pubic and armpit areas in both sexes, while only male sex hormones stimulate facial hair and body hair and may inhibit the growth of some scalp hair. Estrogen stimulates scalp hair.[1]

3. **Nutrition:** Hair follicles must receive a lot of building material to grow hair. A deficiency of certain amino acids, vitamins, and minerals, as well as their malabsorption in the gut, may impair hair growth and cause hair loss.

4. **Emotional distress:** Intense emotional distress such as grief or shock can cause hair loss and premature graying.

5. **Inflammation:** Often linked to stress, inflammation can cause hair follicles to progressively shrink so that they produce thinner and more fragile hair.

6. **Autoimmune diseases:** Alopecia areata is a mysterious disease that causes bald spots or a complete hair loss.

7. **Hormonal problems:** A lack of growth hormone and an imbalance of thyroid hormones may cause hair loss. Some women experience hair loss after pregnancy.

8. **Circulation:** The blood and lymph deliver oxygen and nutrients to the hair, as well as remove toxins. Poor circulation will impair hair growth.

9. **Damage to follicles:** Hair dyes, permanents, straightening, extreme heat, certain ingredients in shampoos, many hair-styling products, tight hairbands, and ultraviolet radiation damage all affect the hair follicles.

10. **Internal diseases and medications:** Hair reflects the overall state of health of the body, therefore digestive issues, hormonal imbalance, liver problems, and autoimmune and inflammatory conditions influence hair's vitality and growth.

TESTOSTERONE AND HAIR LOSS

It was proposed a long time ago that male baldness is somehow linked to male sex hormones, or androgens. Today we know that the male hormone testosterone is indeed responsible for androgenic alopecia, or hair loss. Androgenic alopecia causes characteristic patterns of baldness in men, where the hair either recedes from the front or disappears on the top. Women can also develop this condition, but women rarely go bald and usually experience more diffuse hair loss. For both men and women, hair loss can cause emotional distress. Since emotional distress by itself is capable of causing hair loss, it can further contribute to the problem.

The main culprit in androgenic alopecia is not testosterone itself, but dihydrotestosterone, or DHT, which is produced in the skin and prostate from testosterone by a special enzyme, 5-alpha-reductase.

Testosterone is responsible for masculine characteristics, and DHT is responsible for prostate enlargement, acne, male baldness, and male pattern hair growth. There are two types of 5-alpha reductase: Type 1, which exists predominantly in the skin and liver, and Type 2, which is the major type found in the prostate.[2]

It is not enough to have a high level of DHT in the skin in order to develop androgenic alopecia. In respond to DHT, the hair follicles on the head must have specialized receptors to DHT. Normally, hair follicles are indifferent to male sex hormones. The problem begins when certain scalp hair follicles start responding to DHT by developing DHT receptors. Nobody quite understands how this happens, but it seems to be genetically determined. Once hair follicles start responding to DHT, it shortens their growth phase (anagen) and eventually causes miniaturization (progressive shrinkage) of the hair follicles. As a result, with each hair cycle the hair grows thinner and thinner until the follicles start producing thin, barely visible vellus hair instead of thick, beautiful terminal hair. Men usually have DHT-sensitive hair follicles all grouped together, typically on the forehead and on top of the head. These are the areas where hair loss is often profound and noticeable (male-pattern baldness). In some cases, every single one of the hair follicles on a man's head is DHT-sensitive, eventually resulting in complete baldness.

Women, on the other hand, have a more diffuse distribution of DHT-sensitive follicles. That is why women rarely go completely bald and instead may only develop thinning hair. Since the degree of DHT-dependent hair loss is determined by the DHT sensitivity of the hair follicles, it is quite possible for a man to have a full head of hair regardless of a high level of DHT. People who experience androgenic alopecia may not necessarily have elevated blood testosterone; therefore losing hair and growing bald does not necessarily indicate "superior virility" in a man or a "lack of femininity" in a woman. A receptor to DHT can be compared to a lock that can be only opened with a specific key, which in this case is DHT. If we have the key but there is no lock, the key is useless. This is why even with high testosterone and DHT, a person can have thick, lush hair. If we only have the lock but not the key, the lock won't open. Therefore if DHT-positive hair follicles are present but there is no DHT, the hair will stay thick and healthy. Both the key and the lock have to be present in order for the biological effect to occur. If DHT-positive follicles are near the forehead, that area will grow bald. If these follicles are on the top of the head, then the top of the head will lose hair. If all the follicles on the head have DHT receptors, then eventually the entire head will grow bald.

Male pattern baldness is inherited, going from fathers to sons. Women usually experience only a progressive thinning of their hair, which often occurs in menopause, when declining estrogen levels stop balancing testosterone. Usually thinning hair in menopause is associated with increased hair growth on the face, skin oiliness, and acne due to the increased effects of testosterone.[3]

Androgenic alopecia can be slowed down by the selective inhibitors of 5-alpha reductase. One such remedy is the pharmaceutical drug finasteride, which originally was developed for treating prostate

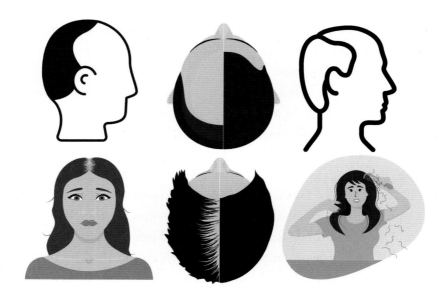

Figure 13.6. Male and female patterns of hair loss in androgenic alopecia.

enlargement in men until it was noticed that it also helps men slow down hair loss. Finasteride does not work for women. For women, bioidentical hormones (i.e., estrogen) can prevent the thinning of hair in menopause. Alternately, phytoestrogens, which are plant compounds found in red clover, nettles, soybeans, pomegranate, and dates, can supply hormones that can help maintain beautiful hair as well as alleviate other symptoms of menopause. Since the skin and fatty tissues are capable of making estrogen, women might want to consider keeping on a little extra weight in menopause, which will help the body make more estrogen. As well, the Taoist practices of using a yoni egg (described in chapter 9) can also help direct sexual energy to the scalp to support the growth of beautiful hair. Retinoic acid (0.01 to 0.05 percent) has also been found to stimulate the hair follicles, helping produce thicker hair shafts.

HAIR UNDER STRESS

Telogen effluvium is the scientific name for hair loss caused by stress. This condition was first described by American dermatologist Albert Kligman in 1961.[4] Some common triggers for telogen effluvium are high fever, major surgery, pregnancy and childbirth, emotional stress, shock, and serious injury. When hair follicles are affected by a triggering event, a large number of them may arrest their growth, enter the telogen phase, and eventually shed hair. It is not clear why some hair follicles are affected and others are not. Most people with telogen effluvium who come to see a dermatologist are women. It's not always easy to identify the triggers for hair loss because with telogen effluvium, noticeable shedding of hair occurs approximately three months after the triggering event. Usually this noticeable thinning resolves after six months, provided the body does not experience more stress, so the main treatment for telogen effluvium is elimination of the stressor (if possible), dedicated self-care, and stress-management techniques.

Postpartum telogen effluvium sometimes coexists with another, opposite condition called *telogen gravidarum,* which occurs when high-circulating estrogen during pregnancy produces a head full of hair. The decline of estrogen in postpartum leads to hair loss, which is physiological and does not require treatment. However, when a woman experiences additional stressing events, such as postpartum depression, relationship issues, or work-related stress, added hair loss due to telogen effluvium may result in noticeable and distressing hair loss and thinning, which sometimes adds more stress and emotional pain.

Telogen effluvium may also be caused by a genetic predisposition to a short anagen phase. In this case, people are unable to grow long hair and are susceptible to hair thinning and hair loss. Another case of sudden hair loss may occur due to treatment with hair growth-stimulating drugs such as minoxidil. In this case, a sudden hair loss is an illusion, caused by many resting follicles awakening from their rest all at once and simultaneously shedding old hair to prepare the way for new hair growth. This may look like sudden hair loss, but in fact it's just a shedding of hair that was already on its way out.

The main recommendations for preventing and alleviating telogen effluvium are building emotional resilience and taking care of negative emotional energy. Inner Smile Chi Kung, described in chapter 4, and Six Healing Sounds Chi Kung, found in chapter 7, are practices that allow for a timely release of stress and negative emotional energy, and a building of positive emotional energy.

HAIR LOSS DUE TO DAMAGE

The longer the hair, the longer it will be subjected to various damaging factors. Newly emerging hair is flexible and strong, and has healthy and resilient cuticles. As long as the cuticles are intact, the hair is smooth, shiny, strong, and can withstand bending and twisting, rain and sunlight, heat and cold. However, hair has one vulnerability: it is held together by the sulfur-rich amino acid cysteine, which forms weak chemical links called *disulfide bonds* between its residues located within the keratin fibrils and the fatty acids in the cuticle. These links work really well until they are exposed to water. So every time you

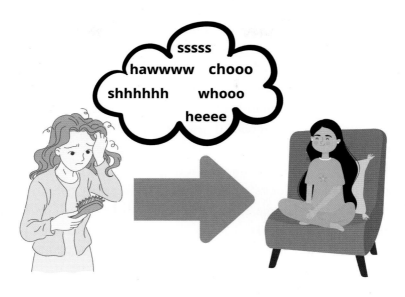

Figure 13.7. Six Healing Sounds Chi Kung helps maintain beautiful hair by preventing stress-related hair loss.

wash your hair with hot (not warm) water and shampoo, which makes the cuticles more permeable, water gets into the hair structure and weakens the links. Once the hair is dry, the links are reestablished. This is why we can make curly hair by wrapping wet hair around curlers and letting it dry. The chemicals used in permanents break the disulfide bonds in the proteins that hold the hair together during the process of wrapping the hair around a roller to form it into a new texture. As a result, the disulfide bonds are chemically reset, and the new, curly texture locks into place. However when the perming solution is left on for too long, is too strong, or when applied to chemically damaged hair, the hair and follicles can get severely damaged. These chemicals also can cause loss of cysteine from the hair, so it becomes spongier and easier to damage. Once the hair cuticles start breaking down, the more fragile cortex is exposed. Eventually, the hair starts breaking and splitting. Since hair cuticles creates shine by reflecting light, and create flexibility of the hair because of the cuticles' lipid coating, a loss of cuticle creates dull, dry, easy-to-tangle hair.

As with perms, the harsh chemicals in straighteners can cause severe damage to the hair. Hair relaxers, typically creams or cream lotions, contain about 2 to 4 percent of strong bases such as sodium hydroxide, potassium hydroxide, and lithium hydroxide, or 5 percent calcium hydroxide plus a solution of up to about 30 percent guanidine carbonate. During the hair straightening procedure, these chemicals break down disulfide bonds in curly hair. It is very important to give hair very good care before and after permanents or relaxers and use a high-quality conditioner to help prevent future damage. It is also recommended that such procedures as perming and straightening be done in a salon, where trained professionals can make sure that your scalp is protected and the solution is not kept on for too long, thereby minimizing the risk of damage.

Once hair emerges from the skin, it cannot be repaired. Yet the hair-care industry keeps enticing people with products that promise to repair, restore, and renew damaged hair. Mostly this results in a temporary improvement (conditioning) by lubricating the hair, changing its shape and flexibility, fortifying it by providing extra coating, and making it softer and shinier. There's nothing wrong with this as long as we remember that in order to help hair grow thicker and stronger, we need to take care of the skin and hair follicles. Good hair conditioners can help protect the hair from external damage such as ultraviolet radiation, dryness, tangles, static electricity, and pollutants. Unfortunately, because the hair-care industry is focused on the external part of the hair, they've created products and procedures that can damage the hair and hair follicles. The rule of thumb is simple: anything that is unhealthy to the skin is also unhealthy for hair follicles. This includes procedures that involve heat, caustic chemicals, chemical dyes, bleach, ammonia, pulling hair, and holding hair in one position for a long time. These influences become even more damaging with age due to declining chi and increased inflammation, especially when combined with other aggravating conditions such as stress, internal illnesses, nutritional imbalance, and already weakened hair.

There are two types of hair loss caused by hair damage. First, breakage of hair strands due to damage to the cuticle and cortex. And second, hair loss caused by damage to the skin and hair follicles. Hair follicles are cradles for hair stem cells. They also harbor a special population of skin stem cells hidden in a special structure called the *hair bulge,* which is a reservoir of stem cells near the skin's surface. When the skin is damaged, stem cells from the bulge migrate into the skin and repair it. Hair follicles are distributed throughout the skin, including the body, so even in the areas that seem hairless there are hair follicles harboring stem cells. Since the bulge is close to the skin's surface, it is vulnerable to toxic, caustic, and irritating substances as well as extreme heat.

Inflammation and poor circulation are common causes of hair loss related to damaging hair treatments. Inflammation causes hair follicles to shorten their growing phase and stay longer in the resting phase. It can also lead to progressive shrinking of the follicles, which produce

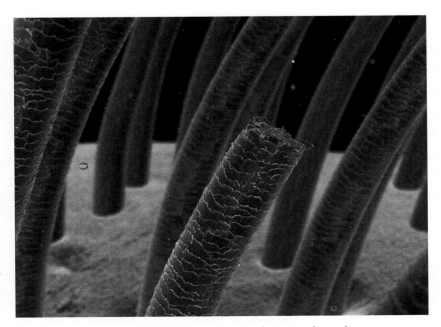

Figure 13.8. Damage to the hair cuticle and cortex causes breakages and hair loss.

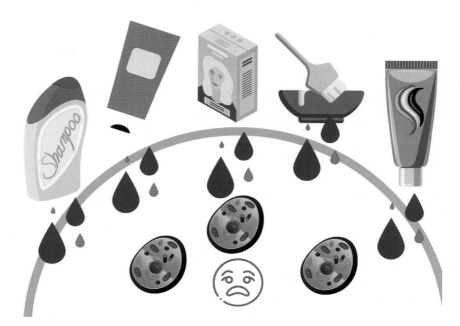

Figure 13.9. Stem cells residing in the hair follicle bulge can be damaged by different types of hair products.

thinner and weaker hair. Inflammation in hair follicles can be triggered by irritating and toxic substances in hair products, allergies, stress, mechanical damage such as pulling, and overheating. All these influences result in a progressive thinning of the hair; brittle and split ends; dry and dull hair; and loss of shine, vitality, and beauty. Even though conditioners can improve the appearance of hair, once the conditioner is washed off, the hair will return to its dismal state. This is why those who want to have thick, luscious, shiny hair need to focus on scalp hair and hair follicles, and if considering a hair treatment, check to see if it is going to help the hair grow or damage it.

Another reason for stunted hair growth and hair loss is lack of hair movement. Hair growing out of hair follicles is held in place by tiny muscles. Just as animals have the ability to bristle when they sense danger, humans too can have a "hair-raising" experience, only not as noticeable. When hair moves, muscles tense and relax, activating blood and lymph flow. So in order to have good microcirculation, hair has to move. Longer hair moves more, and because of its movement and weight, it can build stronger muscles that are better at activating circulation. At the same time, longer hair is more likely to break and entangle. A traditional braid is the ideal hairstyle for long hair providing it is not too tight at the top. As the braid moves with body movement, it activates circulation in the scalp while protecting long strands from breaking. The worst hairstyle for long hair is a hairband, since it can eventually wear out hair cuticles and expose the cortex, making hair vulnerable to breakage. Since shorter hair is lighter and moves even less, it's important for people with short hair to massage their scalp regularly. Hairstyles that keep hair in place, such as strong-hold hairspray that fixes hair in one position, and restrictive hair coverings and wigs that are worn over natural hair for an extended period of time (hours) limit hair movement and impede circulation. If holding hair in one position is necessary, it is important to massage the scalp and let the hair go free whenever possible. When people sit too long without moving, the hair doesn't move as it does when people are walking, running, bending, and stretching. This is why including the

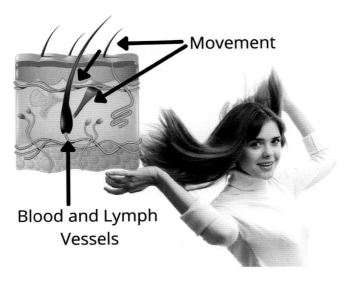

Figure 13.10. Hair movement stimulates blood and lymph flow.

physical movements of Chi Kung in a daily routine helps not only the skin, but also the hair to stay healthy and beautiful.

GRAY AND WHITE HAIR

Hair, like skin, has pigments. This is accomplished by melanocytes, cells that produce granules of the pigment melanin and deposit them in growing hair. With age there are fewer melanocytes in the hair follicles, so the hair gradually becomes less pigmented. Eventually all melanocytes vanish and the hair turns white. At the same time, due to a gradual decline of stem cells, the hair may grow thinner and more sparce. This kind of age-related hair loss is different from hair loss in menopause due to the decline of estrogen. It is important to understand, however, that these kinds of changes are not inevitable, and that gray and white hair can still be thick, healthy, and beautiful provided the scalp and hair follicles are well-maintained, vital, and vibrant.

In both the skin and the hair, melanin protects proteins and lipids from damaging UV radiation by absorbing ultraviolet. When hair is exposed to the sun for a long time, its color fades due to the chemical changes to its melanin. The intermediate products of melanin synthesis are antioxidants that help protect hair follicles from free radicals of oxygen produced in the skin because of UV radiation. Another less well-known function of melanin is its ability to bind to heavy metal ions and some other toxins, which are removed from the skin by growing hair. Since hair itself is not alive, it can serve as a depository for heavy metals and other pollutants. Anyone who lives in a major city carries a periodic table of chemical elements on their head! Hair can tell a story about levels of pollution, lifestyle choices, drug use, and a whole range of health problems. Since gray and white hair lack melanin and therefore cannot remove pollutants from the skin as well as pigmented hair does, special care should be taken to use toxin-free products when one has white and gray hair.

Like all cells, melanocytes undergo natural aging. Their DNA

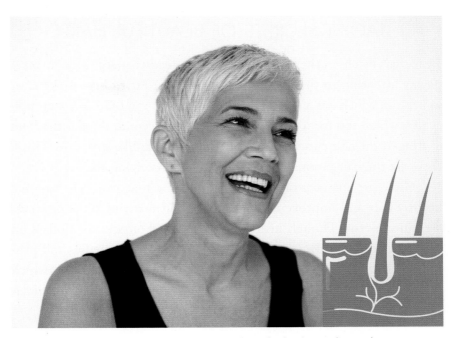

Figure 13.11. Gray and white hair lacks the melanin that normally gives hair its color.

and proteins can be damaged by free radicals of oxygen produced as a result of UV radiation, stress, inflammation, and toxins, all of which can cause premature graying. There is a genetic component in premature hair graying both on the level of inherited genes and epigenetically altered gene expression. Global downregulation of genes responsible for pigmentation has been found in some individuals with premature hair graying.[5]

Protecting hair from UV radiation and using antioxidants can slow down graying. Frequent use of ammonia-based hair dyes, straighteners, perms, and heat, as well as high level of pollutants and stress can accelerate the graying of hair. Hair graying cannot be avoided, but it is possible to have beautiful and healthy gray and white hair. To achieve this, you have to shift your focus—from hiding your gray to loving your gray and honoring it with more dedicated care.

TAOIST SECRETS OF BEAUTIFUL HAIR

By increasing chi in the body, the hair will greatly benefit. This involves paying attention to the various hair structures: First, there is the layer of keratin, which has a crystal-like structure and can bind to water molecules, which too form crystal-like structures. Second, there is the lipid coating of the hair cuticle, which also has a crystal-like structure. Third, there are the hair pores, which are capable of receiving chi.

There are many products on the market that can help support healthy hair and improve its appearance, and many of these products are quite useful. Though many people spend thousands of dollars on hair products, hair dyes, haircuts, and hair-growing remedies and procedures, they still do not have a system of daily hair maintenance, which can make a big difference. The following are a few simple recommendations that do not require expensive hair remedies or procedures.

Tips for Beautiful Hair

- **Bone comb:** Brush your hair daily at least forty to fifty times from the crown down using a bone or horn comb. Taoists traditionally used buffalo horn for a comb. Vegans can use a wooden comb, just make sure it is well-polished and doesn't damage the hair cuticles. It's important to always comb from the base of the scalp to the ends of the hair strands, and never comb wet hair, because the cuticle of the hair is held in place by weak chemical bonds which loosen when hair is wet. This allows curling and styling of wet hair, but also makes wet hair more vulnerable to damage.
- **Scalp massage:** Massage your scalp with your fingers frequently. This will help stimulate circulation to the hair follicles. Stem Cell Chi Kung (described in chapter 6), in which you gently vibrate your scalp with a bamboo hitter, also works to stimulate blood flow.
- **Gentle cleansing:** It is important to wash your hair with warm water only (not hot) and select a mild shampoo. A good-quality

conditioner will help protect your hair from damage and make it more manageable and flexible.

- **Healing love:** In menopause, when scalp skin starts receiving less estrogen, Taoists recommended moving one's sexual energy from the sexual organs to the head through the practices of Healing Love Chi Kung, such as those described in chapter 9 of this book, and the Microcosmic Orbit Meditation described in chapter 8. Sexual energy is like water in that like the water that helps trees grow it similarly stimulates regeneration and growth of hair. When combined with unconditional love, this produces a healing elixir that stimulates the stem cells and improves hair growth.

- **Relax and release:** Inner Smile Chi Kung, found in chapter 4, and the Six Healing Sounds Chi Kung, found in chapter 7, allow you to release negative emotions, relax the body, and alleviate stress.

- **Movement:** Physical exercises must be done regularly to move scalp hair and bring more blood, oxygen, nutrients, and moisture to hair follicles.

- **Nutritional support:** Eating vibrant food containing the colors of the five elements as described in chapter 12 helps supply the skin with important nutrients such as copper, zinc, sulfur, vitamins, essential amino acids, phytoestrogens, and omega 3 fatty acids, all of which support hair growth.

- **Hair breathing:** Breathing chi into the hair, described below, activates the hair follicles and helps bring more life force into the body.

- **Gray hair needs more care:** Taoist masters generally live long and healthy lives, coming to great wisdom later in life. Just as the skin and body need more care as we age, gray hair has to be treated with reverence and extra care.

Hair Breathing

1. Sit straight on the edge of a chair or stand in Chi Kung stance, feet hip-width apart, knees slightly bent. Feel your feet connecting to the earth, growing deep roots. Feel your crown connecting to the

cosmos by extending your hair "antennae." Keep your spine straight. Feel your tailbone extending down into the ground.

2. Become aware of your hair. Smile into your hair. Take a deep breath into your nose and let it out through your nose again. On the next inhalation, visualize and feel breathing into your hair and then exhale imagining you are breathing out from your hair.

3. Imagine your hairs extending from your scalp with every breath, like antennae. Inhale golden light into your hair; exhale dark and cloudy energy.

4. Begin abdominal breathing. Inhale, expanding your abdomen. Exhale, moving the navel toward your spine. Repeat nine times.

5. Inhale, then exhale, pulling the navel toward your spine, then hold your breath. As you hold your breath, start pulling your perineum and diaphragm up while imagining you are drawing chi all the way up into the ends of your hair. Inhale, exhale, and relax and rest. Repeat this step nine times.

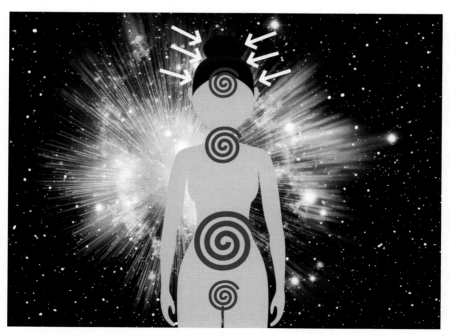

Figure 13.13. Hair breathing tells the mind to use hair as an antenna for chi.

6. Rest, relax, and breathe softly. Smile into your hair.

7. Gently tap your crown and your third eye to activate nerve endings. Now repeat abdominal breathing (described in step 4 above) nine times. Next, inhale, then exhale, holding your breath, and "breathe without breathing" by moving your perineum and diaphragm up. Imagine receiving universal violet light into your crown and your third eye. Let the violet light saturate your brain and scalp.

8. Relax, rest, and breathe through your hair, becoming aware of chi flow.

9. Focus on your navel. Guide chi from your navel into your perineum. Then inhale, pull up your perineum, and guide chi with your eyes, breathing and smiling up the tailbone and sacrum into the Microcosmic Orbit as described in chapter 8.

10. Rest, relax, and smile into your hair.

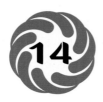

Beauty Chi Kung for Youthful Skin at Any Age

To create radiant skin it is vital to understand that skin is much more than a physical covering for the body. As a living, breathing organ that radiates personal energy and connects the body to nature's energies, the skin is what makes us feel alive. Tingling, buzzing, warm sensations add a delightful richness to exciting experiences, while chills and goose-bumps make a scary movie even more thrilling. The skin can keep us safe, like a radiant shield, or it can keep failing us, like a broken fence that is neither beautiful nor functional. The skin can radiate our inner beauty or reveal our insecurities and unhealthy lifestyle. Skin beauty is more than skin-deep, and it can tell more tales than people realize.

The Tao teaches that the skin is the largest organ, that which connects us to the universe. It is the territory between the interior of the body and the outside environment. And just like at any borderland, the skin has to control what enters and what must be rejected. It has to sense the energy in the outer environment and respond appropriately. When the skin is blocked, energy cannot flow. Taoist masters traditionally pay careful attention to the condition of their skin. According to the Tao, the skin has to be clean, youthful, and healthy at any age in

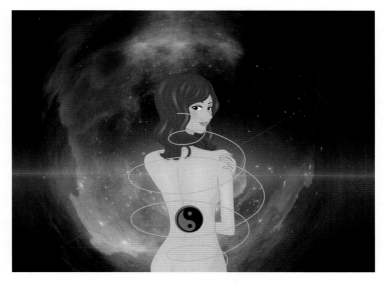

Figure 14.1. Energy flows between the skin and the universe.

order to serve as a bridge and interface between the body and the universe. When the skin stops taking in energy and stops radiating light, there is no beauty and no life.

BEAUTIFUL SKIN IS AGELESS

The Taoist idea of skin beauty is very different from what most westerners believe. In the West, beautiful skin has become a myth, an illusion, something attainable only by a few rare persons. Inspired by poets and advertisements, this myth makes people chase an impossible ideal of eternally young and flawless skin. In reality, the skin may be far from ideal. Even famous models who wow us with their flawless faces often have to mask their imperfections with carefully applied makeup and artful lighting. Today, with the advent of artificial intelligence, presenting an impossibly perfect image of eternal youth has become even easier.

From adolescent skin, with its excessive oiliness, enlarged pores, and acne, to mature skin, with its wrinkles, pigment spots, scars, and other imperfections, the skin is a record of our life experiences and choices as it responds to negative emotions, poor nutrition, a polluted environment, and biological aging. When people experience frustration over their skin imperfections, they may waste a lot of money and energy on desperate attempts to achieve an impossible ideal. Paradoxically, many of these efforts may do more harm than good, causing a person to choose products and procedures that promise fast and impressive results, but are actually harmful. Products loaded with synthetic chemicals, including texture stabilizers, emulsifiers, lubricants, preservatives, colorants, and artificial fragrance may create the illusion of beautification, but if used for too long they will block the skin's chi and cause it to lose its vitality.

It's time to rethink what it means to have beautiful skin, because standard definitions exclude those whose skin reflects all the ups and downs of the rich life a person has lived. Once we realize that truly beautiful skin is skin that is healthy, vibrant, radiant, and sensual, connected to nature's energies and radiating one's inner light and individuality, it becomes clear that beautiful skin is attainable at any age,

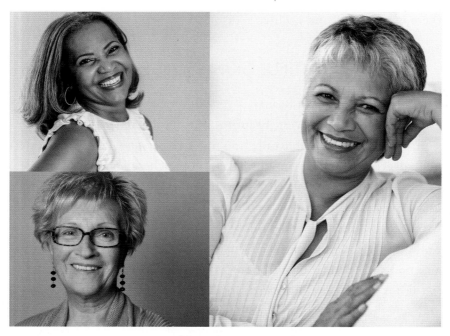

Figure 14.2. It is possible to have radiant skin as we mature.

regardless of physical characteristics. Beautiful skin is eternal and timeless, and its attraction is not diminished by biological age.

BEAUTY CARE IS CHI CARE

Beauty Chi Kung is a time-tested practice that takes into account the skin's connection to the body, mind, soul, spirit, and universe. Today modern science confirms what ancient Taoist masters have been teaching for thousands of years: it is not enough to take care of the skin physically; it is vital that we take care of its energy, or chi, as well. However it is also not enough to take care of the chi in the skin only, because the energy of the skin does not function independently; it is an integral part of the flow of energy of the entire body, physically attached to the body through layers of muscle, fat, and connective tissue, as well as through the nerves, blood vessels, and lymphatic vessels. The skin transmits chi and connects all parts of the body through a web of energy channels. Therefore taking care of the body means taking care of the skin, and taking care of the skin means taking care of the body.

Five Essential Jobs Your Skin Cannot Do Alone

1. **Digestion and absorption:** To be beautiful, the skin has to repair and regenerate. To repair and regenerate, the skin needs nutrients. The skin does not have teeth or its own digestive system, so it needs the body to chew, swallow, and digest food. It then needs the heart and blood vessels to deliver nutrients to the cells.

2. **Elimination of toxins:** Beautiful skin needs to be clean and free of toxins. The skin can eliminate some toxins and CO_2, but it still needs the lungs, kidneys, and liver to remove the bulk of CO_2, toxins, and metabolites.

3. **Breathing:** To be beautiful and resilient, the skin needs oxygen to make chi. The skin doesn't have its own lungs, and even though it can absorb some oxygen from the air, it still needs the rest of the body to breathe oxygen and release CO_2.

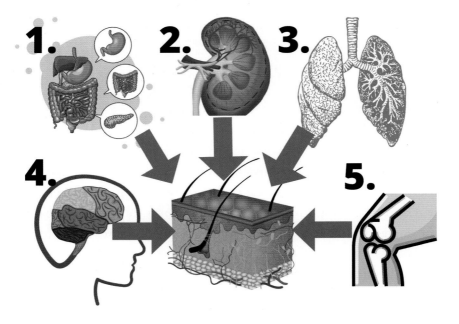

Figure 14.3. Five jobs the skin cannot do alone.

4. **Protection:** The skin does not have eyes and cannot watch out for sharp edges and thorns. So it needs the eyes, ears, and the body's nervous system to perceive dangers and pleasures in the environment. The flow of emotions triggered by the senses energizes and enlivens the skin. Beautiful skin also needs protection from viruses, bacteria, parasites, and other invaders. The skin has its own emergency response team, but when it comes to dealing with disasters, it needs help from the entire body.

5. **Mechanical support:** The skin needs fat, muscles, ligaments, fascia, and bones to support its weight and give it shape. When the underlying structure weakens, the skin sags.

Each of these tasks can be quite daunting if we attempt to solve them separately. However, there is no need to address every system individually. The skin and body are quite capable of regulating themselves as long as they are connected through the flow of bioelectromagnetic energy. Beauty Chi Kung works with the river of chi that flows through the organs, tissues, and cells. The invisible flow of chi fills the skin with life, radiance, and beauty. Chi is life flowing through the skin and through all living things. The difference between electricity that illuminates our houses and powers up our cellphones and electricity that animates our skin is that the skin needs *bioelectromagnetic* energy, which can only be produced by living cells, which themselves need energy to make energy. It takes chi to make chi. It takes life to create more life.

Ancient Taoists developed powerful energy practices and honed them over thousands of years, carefully transmitting them from masters to novices. They realized that in order to recharge and replenish our body's biological batteries, all the organs need to work in harmony. There is no such thing as "just the skin" or "just the heart"; all organs work as an integrated whole. Healthy lungs can take in more oxygen, while a healthy heart and blood vessels can more efficiently deliver blood to skin cells. A robust and healthy capillary network in the skin not only infuses it with a radiant, healthy glow, it is also more efficient at bringing oxygen to every cell and removing toxic CO_2 before it gets absorbed into the skin tissue. A healthy gut can digest and absorb nutrients much better compared to an inflamed, constipated, or leaky gut. Every step in the process of energy production depends on the health and coordinated work of trillions of cells, and the healthier they are, the more chi will flow to the skin, and the more radiant and beautiful it will look. Every organ in the body contributes to producing chi for the skin's needs. This is why happy organs working in harmony under optimal conditions can help us achieve beautiful and radiant skin.

A healthy young person has vibrant, resilient, beautiful skin. However when people continue to spend their chi the way they did when they were young, they are behaving like an ex-billionaire who no longer has their billions yet cannot let go of their luxury spending habits. In the hard-driving West there is an epidemic of burnout. When

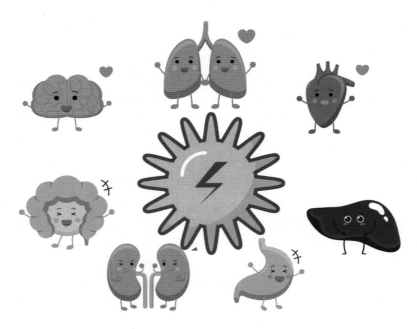

Figure 14.4. Happy organs working in harmony make more chi.

chi is very low, the body will have difficulty resisting infections, digesting and absorbing food, and detoxing and balancing hormones. This is reflected in the skin, which loses its radiance. Wise people watch their spending even when they are enjoying good fortune; in the same way it's very important to know how to replenish one's own energy fortune of chi so as not to go broke.

Beauty Chi Kung is the missing ingredient in skin care because it addresses the most essential need of the skin: the generation of chi. While we can recharge our phone by plugging it into an electrical outlet, such an option is not available to our body. But this does not mean that the body does not have to be recharged. Every living organism has to be able to replenish its bioelectromagnetic energy, otherwise it will deplete itself and die. A strong, healthy body can make more chi compared to a weak, sick, depleted body. So a strong and healthy body can perform better and have more radiance, more resilience, and more stamina.

In addition to the bioelectromagnetic energy that animates all the cells and tissues, the skin is also strongly influenced by the bioelectromagnetic energy of our thoughts, emotions, and spiritual essence. Therefore mind, body, and spirit work together to create beautiful and radiant skin. The emotions move the skin and alter its physiology through changes in muscle tension, blood flow, immune reactivity, oxygen availability, temperature, and chemistry. This is why releasing negative emotions and replenishing with positive energy is an essential daily practice to achieving beautiful skin and a healthy body.

Beauty Chi Kung as described in this book is a complete mind/body/spirit practice. It involves simple, enjoyable, powerful practices for preserving, enhancing, and restoring the skin's beauty. When organized into a meaningful daily routine or ritual, Beauty Chi Kung becomes a part of life, the same as taking a daily shower and brushing one's teeth.

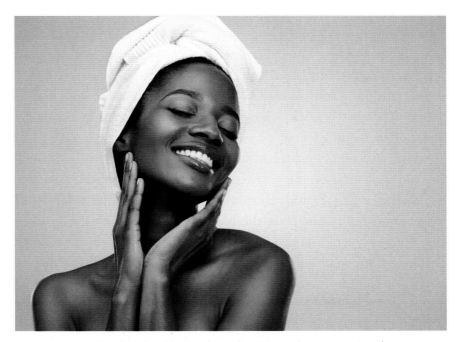

Figure 14.5. A healthy body makes more chi, creating radiant and beautiful skin.

DEVELOPING YOUR BEAUTY PRACTICE

The best way to start practicing Beauty Chi Kung is to set aside thirty minutes for your daily protocol. Since Beauty Chi Kung improves energy flow throughout the entire body, your whole life will benefit from these practices. Soon, Beauty Chi Kung will be a natural and easy part of your routine. You do not need to do all the practices every day. When you have more time, do more. When you have less time, do less. Make it interesting by varying your practice. As your energy level and health improves, and your skin starts radiating balanced, clean, clear, nourishing energy, you will start enjoying your practices and will want to do more.

Morning Practice

Upon awakening in the morning, don't jump out of the bed right away. It's important to let the body adjust to a waking state. This is a good time to smile into all your organs and skin, sending them gratitude and love. Taoist Healing Love practices such as breast massage and yoni egg practices, described in chapter 9, can be done right after taking a shower or during your shower. It is important to massage your breasts before starting your work day, especially for women who spend all day in the office wearing a bra.

After brushing your teeth, taking a shower, and getting dressed, you can do your morning practice. It's a good habit to start your day by drinking a glass of pure, clean water. During sleep, the kidneys still work, removing toxins from the blood, so if you don't drink water first thing in the morning, a lot of toxins will get stuck in the kidneys. Drinking water helps flush them out once you start moving. However avoid drinking too much water in the morning as you don't want to overburden your kidneys. One glass is enough.

Choices of morning exercises are the Inner Smile (chapter 4), physical movements of Chi Kung, Skin Breathing (chapter 5), and Iron Shirt Chi Kung (chapter 10). This will activate skin circulation and make you look more confident, beautiful, and radiant. Also, because these practices improve the overall flow of energy, you may notice that you have more focus, clearer thinking, more energy, greater motivation, and a more relaxed attitude toward life.

Morning is the best time to apply a quality moisturizer. Apply it to slightly damp skin to help preserve moisture. Your daily moisturizer has to contain antioxidants to protect the skin from pollution and UV radiation.

Taoist masters discovered that there are times when chi flows more to some organs than to others. Focusing on these times helps direct more flow to the organs that need chi. The timetable for chi flow to the organs is as follows: During breakfast, remember to chew your food until it's liquid, and add good chi to your meal by imagining a beautiful place or looking at a picture of a beautiful place and sending gratitude to your meal, the planet, and all those who helped put this food on the table. Notice the colors and vibrancy of your food. Soon you will intuitively include foods that have the colors of the five elements. The

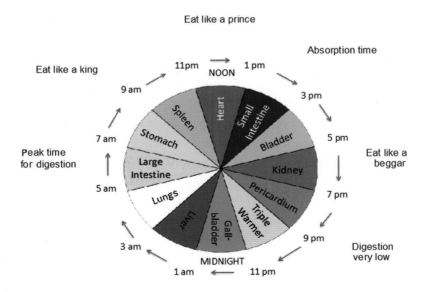

Figure 14.6. Timetable for chi flow to the organs.

more you connect to your food energetically, the more your body will activate its innate wisdom. Many people report reaching their weight goals naturally this way, without dieting.

During the Day

If you drive to work there are some practices you can do in the car. One of them is squeezing and releasing your perineum to send a flow of radiant energy up your spine. It doesn't require much time and can be done safely while waiting in traffic or waiting for the traffic light to change.

The more you spread your practice throughout your day, the more practice you can fit in, and the more creative you will become in fitting more practices in. The proper time to massage your breasts is right after you come home from work and can take your bra off.

Evening Practice

It's important to not practice too close to bedtime, or it may make it more difficult to fall asleep. The only exception is Six Healing Sounds Chi Kung (chapter 7), which encourages relaxation and allows us to let go of daily stress before sleep. Evening is the best time to apply skin products that contain biologically active ingredients that stimulate repair and regeneration. They will work while you sleep and rest. Scrubs, peels, and other exfoliating products are also better to use before sleep. Remember to protect your skin from the UV radiation the next morning after exfoliation. Smile into your skin when you apply skincare products. Imagine sending good energy to your skin.

BEAUTY CHI KUNG FOR LIFE

It's important to remember that just as with skin-care products, when you start practicing Beauty Chi Kung you'll notice an immediate improvement in the skin's radiance and beauty, and there are also delayed effects that will appear weeks or even months later. The skin is a living organ, and it takes time to replenish, rebalance, and rejuvenate. It's also important to remember that even though the body and every organ in it ages with each passing day, there are also antiaging processes that involve the repair, regeneration, and removal of damaging structures, and the healing of damaged tissues. The more we can protect the skin from factors that accelerate its aging, and the more we can help our own natural antiaging processes, the more young, healthy, and beautiful the skin will look.

Beauty is more than vanity. It's possible to see the effects of an unhealthy lifestyle and internal illness by observing the skin. Often the skin is the first organ that indicates an internal problem. The skin is a tale-telling organ. The more we care about its beauty from a holistic perspective, the more the entire body benefits. The same way, processing our negative emotions and not blocking or suppressing them will help the skin and the entire body. A healthy, balanced, clean and clear mind can better regulate the cells and organs. Reducing stress helps reduce inflammation and restores good digestion. Cultivating beauty, therefore, can be the guiding light that helps a person take a better care of their body, mind, and spirit.

As Taoist wisdom teaches, a good heart, a good mind, and good chi brings long life, good health, and good luck. The quest for beauty can become a spiritual journey that will keep bringing new discoveries, new gifts, and new happiness to enjoy and share with others. Start where you are. Start with baby steps. Do what you can, but do it daily. Celebrate small victories. Remember to smile. And watch your skin becoming more beautiful, radiant, and alive.

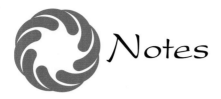# Notes

Introduction.
Why Beauty Products Don't Work

1. Chris Kolmar, "24 Powerful Cosmetics Industry Statistics [2023]: What's Trending in the Beauty Business?" Zippia website, March 2, 2023.
2. Waly Fall and Céline Trophardy, "Effets du maquillage sur l'humeur et la marche chez la femme âgée" [Effects of makeup on mood and walking in elderly women], *Soins* 66, no. 859 (2021): 34–38.
3. N. Leigh-Hunt et al., "An Overview of Systematic Reviews on the Public Health Consequences of Social Isolation and Loneliness," *Public Health* 152 (November 2017): 157–71.
4. A. Pourang et al., "Effects of Visible Light on Mechanisms of Skin Photoaging," *Photodermatology, Photoimmunology, and Photomedicine* 38, no. 3 (May 2022): 191–96.
5. H. W. Lim et al., "Impact of Visible Light on Skin Health: The Role of Antioxidants and Free Radical Quenchers in Skin Protection," *Journal of the American Academy of Dermatology* 86, no. 3S (2022): S27–S37.
6. S. Cho et al., "Effects of Infrared Radiation and Heat on Human Skin Aging In Vivo," *Journal of Investigative Dermatology Symposium Proceedings* 14, no. 1 (2009): 15–19.
7. A. Vierkötter and J. Krutmann, "Environmental Influences on Skin Aging and Ethnic-Specific Manifestations," *Dermato-Endocrinology* 4, no. 3 (2012): 227–31; C. Parrado et al., "Environmental Stressors on Skin Aging: Mechanistic Insights," *Frontiers in Pharmacology* 10 (2019): 759.
8. Wan-Lin Teo, "The 'Maskne' Microbiome—Pathophysiology and Therapeutics," *International Journal of Dermatology* 60, no. 7 (2021): 799–809.

9. A. R. Darnall, D. Sall, and C. Bay, "Types and Prevalence of Adverse Skin Reactions Associated with Prolonged N95 and Simple Mask Usage during the COVID-19 Pandemic," *Journal of the European Academy of Dermatology and Venereology* 36, no. 10 (2022): 1805–10; R. D. Jobanputra et al., "A Numerical Analysis of Skin-PPE Interaction to Prevent Facial Tissue Injury," *Scientific Reports* 11, no. 1 (2021): 16248.

10. Y. Chen and J. Lyga, "Brain-Skin Connection: Stress, Inflammation and Skin Aging," *Inflammation and Allergy Drug Targets* 13, no. 3 (2014): 177–90; P. Oyetakin-White et al., "Does Poor Sleep Quality Affect Skin Ageing?" *Clinical and Experimental Dermatology* 40, no. 1 (2015): 17–22.

11. Q. Y. A. Wong and F. T. Chew, "Defining Skin Aging and Its Risk Factors: A Systematic Review and Meta-analysis," *Scientific Reports* 11, no. 1 (2021): 22075.

12. R. Jahnke et al., "A Comprehensive Review of Health Benefits of Qigong and Tai Chi," *American Journal of Health Promotion* 24, no. 6 (2010): e1–e25; B. F. Toneti et al., "Benefits of Qigong as an Integrative and Complementary Practice for Health: A Systematic Review," *Revista Latino-Americana de Enfermagem* 28 (2020): e3317; B. H. Ng and H. W. Tsang, "Psychophysiological Outcomes of Health Qigong for Chronic Conditions: A Systematic Review," *Psychophysiology* 46, no. 2 (2009): 257–69.

13. P. S. Chang et al., "Physical and Psychological Health Outcomes of Qigong Exercise in Older Adults: A Systematic Review and Meta-Analysis," *American Journal of Chinese Medicine* 47, no. 2 (2019): 301–22.

14. S. Agrigoroaei, A. Lee-Attardo, and M. E. Lachman, "Stress and Subjective Age: Those with Greater Financial Stress Look Older," *Research on Aging* 39, no. 10 (2017): 1075–99.

Chapter 1.
Beauty Is More Than Skin-Deep

1. M. M. Hamilton and R. Kao, "Recognizing and Managing Complications in Laser Resurfacing, Chemical Peels, and Dermabrasion," *Facial Plastic Surgery Clinics of North America* 28 no. 4 (November 2020):493–501.

2. Zoe Draelos and Peter T. Pugliese, *Physiology of the Skin,* 3rd Ed. (Carol Stream, Ill.: Allured Publishing, 2011), 7.

3. M. Richardson, "Understanding the Structure and Function of the Skin," *Nursing Times* 99, no. 31 (2003): 46–48.

4. Zoe Draelos and Peter T. Pugliese, *Physiology of the Skin, 3rd Ed.* (Carol Stream, Ill.: Allured Publishing, 2011), 7.

Chapter 2.
Taoist Secrets of Vitality and Vibrancy

1. R. Farahzadi et al., "Targeting the Stem Cell Niche Micro-environment as Therapeutic Strategies in Aging," *Frontiers in Cell and Developmental Biology* 11 (May 19, 2023); Y. Ge et al., "The Aging Skin Microenvironment Dictates Stem Cell Behavior," *PNAS* 117, no. 10 (March 10, 2020): 5339–50.

2. L. C. Matos et al., "Qigong as a Traditional Vegetative Biofeedback Therapy: Long-Term Conditioning of Physiological Mind-Body Effects," *Biomed Research International* (2015).

3. Michael D. Gershon, *The Second Brain: The Scientific Basis of Gut Instinct and a Groundbreaking New Understanding of Nervous Disorders of the Stomach and Intestine* (Harper, 1999).

Chapter 3.
The Yin and Yang of Skin Renewal

1. C. Franceschi et al., "Inflamm-aging: An Evolutionary Perspective on Immunosenescence," *Annals of the New York Academy of Sciences* 908 (2000): 244–54.

Chapter 5.
Breathing Life into Skin

1. Johnjoe McFadden, "The Conscious Electromagnetic Information (Cemi) Field Theory," *Journal of Consciousness Studies* 9, no. 8 (2002): 45–60.

2. F. Vazza and A. Feletti, "The Quantitative Comparison Between the Neuronal Network and the Cosmic Web," *Frontiers in Physics* 8 (2020).

3. A. Farhadi et al., "Evidence for Non-chemical, Non-electrical Intercellular Signaling in Intestinal Epithelial Cells," *Bioelectrochemistry* 71 no. 2 (November 2007):142–48.

Chapter 7.
Beauty and Emotions

1. Andrzej Slominski and Jacobo Wortsman, "Neuroendocrinology of the Skin," *Endocrine Reviews* 21, no. 5 (2000): 457–87; P. L. Bigliardi et al., "Opioids and the Skin—Where Do We Stand?" *Experimental Dermatology* 18, no. 5 (2009): 424–30.

2. W. P. Bowe and A. C. Logan, "Acne vulgaris, Probiotics and the Gut-Brain-Skin Axis: Back to the Future?" *Gut Pathogens* 3, no. 1 (2011).

3. Michael D. Gershon and Kara Gross Margolis, "The Gut, Its Microbiome, and the Brain: Connections and Communications," *Journal of Clinical Investigation* 131 no. 18 (September 2021): e143768.

4. Sigrid Breit et al., "Vagus Nerve as Modulator of the Brain-Gut Axis in Psychiatric and Inflammatory Disorders," *Frontiers in Psychiatry* 9 no. 44 (March 2018).

5. B. E. Kok et al., "How Positive Emotions Build Physical Health: Perceived Positive Social Connections Account for the Upward Spiral between Positive Emotions and Vagal Tone," *Psychological Science* 24, no. 7 (2013): 1123–32.

6. Bruno Bonaz, Thomas Bazin, and Sonia Pellissier, "The Vagus Nerve at the Interface of the Microbiota-Gut-Brain Axis," *Frontiers in Neuroscience* 12 no. 49 (February 2018).

7. Chaoren Tan et al., "Recognizing the Role of the Vagus Nerve in Depression from Microbiota-Gut Brain Axis," *Frontiers in Neurology* 13 (November 2022): 1015175.

8. Tracey Bear et al., "The Microbiome-Gut-Brain Axis and Resilience to Developing Anxiety or Depression under Stress," *Microorganisms* 9 no. 4 (March 2021): 723.

9. Oliver Cameron Reddy and Ysbrand van der Werf, "The Sleeping Brain: Harnessing the Power of the Glymphatic System through Lifestyle Choices," *Brain Sciences* 10 no. 11 (November 2020): 868; Helene Benveniste et al., "The Glymphatic System and Waste Clearance with Brain Aging: A Review," *Gerontology* 65 no. 2 (2019): 106–19.

Chapter 8.
Preserving Youthful Beauty with the Microcosmic Orbit

1. C. M. Chuong et al., "What Is the 'True' Function of Skin?" *Experimental Dermatology* 11 no. 2 (April 2002):159–87.

2. A. Slominski, "A Nervous Breakdown in the Skin: Stress and the Epidermal Barrier," Journal of Clinical Investigation 117 no. 11 (November 2007): 3166–69.

3. L. Marek-Jozefowicz et al., "The Brain-Skin Axis in Psoriasis—Psychological, Psychiatric, Hormonal, and Dermatological Aspects." International Journal of Molecular Sciences 23 no. 2 (January 2022): 669.

4. T. L. Goldsby and M. E. Goldsby, "Eastern Integrative Medicine and Ancient Sound Healing Treatments for Stress: Recent Research Advances," *Integrative Medicine* 19 no. 6 (December 2020): 24–30.

5. This meta-analysis analyzed English, Portuguese, and Spanish language articles published between 2005 and 2015: L. J. Moraes et al., "A Systematic Review of Psychoneuroimmunology-Based Interventions," *Psychology, Health, and Medicine* 23, no. 6 (2018): 635–52.

6. D. Atkinson et al., "A New Bioinformatics Paradigm for the Theory, Research, and Practice of Therapeutic Hypnosis," *American Journal of Clinical Hypnosis* 53 no. 1 (July 2010): 27–46.

7. H. Y. Weng et al., "Interventions and Manipulations of Interoception." Trends in Neurosciences," 44 no. 1 (January 2021): 52–62.

8. C. Coffey and P. O'Leary, "The Mesentery: Structure, Function, and Role in Disease," *The Lancet* 1 no. 3 (2016): 238–47.

9. Mantak Chia and William U. Wei, *Basic Practices of the Universal Healing Tao: An Illustrated Guide to Levels 1 through 6* (Rochester, Vt.: Destiny, 2013).

Chapter 9.
Sexual Energy for Cultivation of Beauty

1. Mantak Chia and Andrew Jan. *The Practice of Greater Kan and Li: Techniques for Creating the Immortal Self.*

2. D. L. Hemsell et al., "Plasma Precursors of Estrogen. II. Correlation of the Extent of Conversion of Plasma Androstenedione to Estrone with Age," *Journal of Clinical Endocrinology and Metabolism* 38 no. 3 (March 1974): 476–79.

3. R. Barakat et al., "Extra-gonadal Sites of Estrogen Biosynthesis and Function," *BMB Reports* 49 no. 9 (September 2016): 488–96.

4. M. C. Canivenc-Lavier, and C. Bennetau-Pelissero, "Phytoestrogens and Health Effects," *Nutrients.* 15 no. 2 (January 2023): 317.

5. Kirsty M. Mair, Rosemary Gaw, and Margaret R. MacLean, "Obesity, Estrogens and Adipose Tissue Dysfunction: Implications for Pulmonary Arterial Hypertension," *Pulmonary Circulation* 10 no. 3 (July–September 2020).

Chapter 10.
Iron Shirt Chi Kung to Maintain Strength and Beauty

1. Xiujie Ma and George Jennings, "'Hang the Flesh off the Bones': Cultivating an 'Ideal Body' in Taijiquan and Neigong," *International Journal of Environ-*

mental Research and Public Health 18 no. 9 (April 2021): 4417; Z. Peng, R. Xu, and Q. You, "Role of Traditional Chinese Medicine in Bone Regeneration and Osteoporosis," *Frontiers in Bioengineering and Biotechnology* 10 (May 2022): 911326; Y. Zhou et al., "Different Training Durations and Frequencies of Tai Chi for Bone Mineral Density Improvement: A Systematic Review and Meta-Analysis." *Evidence-Based Complementary and Alternative Medicine* (March 2021): 6665642.

2. C. S. Colón-Emeric and K. G. Saag, "Osteoporotic Fractures in Older Adults," *Best Practice and Research: Clinical Rheumatology* 20 no. 4 (August 2006): 695–706.

3. "Epidemiology of Osteoporosis and Fragility Fractures," International Osteoporosis Foundation website, accessed August 16, 2023.

4. Pascual-Fernández J. et al., "Sarcopenia: Molecular Pathways and Potential Targets for Intervention." *International Journal of Molecular Science* 21 no. 22 (November 2020): 8844.

5. M. L. Maltais, J. Desroches, and I. J. Dionne, "Changes in Muscle Mass and Strength after Menopause," *Journal of Musculoskeletal and Neuronal Interactions* 9 no. 4 (October–December 2009): 186–97.

6. M. Herrmann et al., "Interactions between Muscle and Bone: Where Physics Meets Biology," *Biomolecules* 10 no. 3 (March 2020): 432.

7. L. Bonewald, "Use It or Lose It to Age: A Review of Bone and Muscle Communication," *Bone* 120 (March 2019): 212–18.

8. W. Sun, X. A. Zhang, and Z. Wang, "The Role and Regulation Mechanism of Chinese Traditional Fitness Exercises on the Bone and Cartilage Tissue in Patients with Osteoporosis: A Narrative Review," *Frontiers in Physiology* 14 (February 2023): 1071005.

9. J. E. Compston et al., "Relationship of Weight, Height, and Body Mass Index with Fracture Risk at Different Sites in Postmenopausal Women: the Global Longitudinal Study of Osteoporosis in Women (GLOW)," *Journal of Bone and Mineral Research* 29 no. 2 (February 2014): 487–93.

10. L. R. Nelson and S. E. Bulun, "Estrogen Production and Action," *Journal of the American Academy of Dermatology* 45 no. 3 (September 2001): S116–24.

11. L. A. Schaap et al., "Inflammatory Markers and Loss of Muscle Mass (Sarcopenia) and Strength," *American Journal of Medicine* 119 no. 6 (June 2006): 526. e9-17.

12. L. Bonewald, "Use It or Lose It to Age: A Review of Bone and Muscle Communication," *Bone* 120 (March 2019): 212–18.

13. C. Stefanaki, P. Pervanidou, D. Boschiero, and G. P. Chrousos. "Chronic Stress and Body Composition Disorders: Implications for Health and Disease." *Hormones* 17 no. 1 (March 2018 Mar): 33–43.

14. Bradley D. Lloyd et al., "Recurrent and Injurious Falls in the Year Following Hip Fracture: A Prospective Study of Incidence and Risk Factors from the Sarcopenia and Hip Fracture Study," *Journals of Gerontology Series A: Biological and Medical Sciences* 64, no. 5 (2009): 599–609.

15. E. Grazioli et al., "Physical Activity in the Prevention of Human Diseases: Role of Epigenetic Modifications," *BMC Genomics* 18 no. 8 (November 2017): 802.

16. Mantak Chia, *Iron Shirt Chi Kung* (Rochester, Vt.: Destiny Books, 2006).

Chapter 11.
Common Skin Problems

1. J. A. Nichols and S. K. Katiyar. "Skin Photoprotection by Natural Polyphenols: Anti-inflammatory, Antioxidant and DNA Repair Mechanisms." *Archives of Dermatological Research* 302 no. 2 (March 2010): 71–83.

2. Z. Tang et al., "Research Progress of Keratinocyte-Programmed Cell Death in UV-Induced Skin Photodamage," *Photodermatology, Photoimmunology, and Photomedicine* 37 no. 5 (September 2021): 442–48.

3. P. Autier, "Sunscreen Abuse for Intentional Sun Exposure," *British Journal of Dermatology* 161 no. 3 (November 2009 Nov): 40–45.

4. S. P. Paul, "Ensuring the Safety of Sunscreens, and Their Efficacy in Preventing Skin Cancers: Challenges and Controversies for Clinicians, Formulators, and Regulators," *Frontiers in Medicine* 6 (September 2019): 195.

5. H. Lee, Y. Hong, and M. Kim, "Structural and Functional Changes and Possible Molecular Mechanisms in Aged Skin," *International Journal of Molecular Sciences* 22 no. 22 (November 2021): 12489.

6. A. Napolitano et al., "Pheomelanin-Induced Oxidative Stress: Bright and Dark Chemistry Bridging Red Hair Phenotype and Melanoma," *Pigment Cell Melanoma Research* 27 no. 5 (September 2014): 721–33.

7. M. Brenner and V. J. Hearing, "The Protective Role of Melanin against UV Damage in Human Skin," *Photochemistry and Photobiology* 84 no. 3 (May–June 2008): 539–49.

8. I. Jozic et al., "Skin under the (Spot)-Light: Cross-Talk with the Central Hypothalamic-Pituitary-Adrenal (HPA) Axis." *Journal of Investigative Dermatology* 135 no. 6 (June 2015): 1469–71.

9. N. Puizina-Ivić, "Skin Aging," *Acta Dermatovenerol Alp Pannonica Adriat.* 17 no. 2 (June 2008): 47–54; T. M. Ansary et al., "Inflammatory Molecules Associated with Ultraviolet Radiation-Mediated Skin Aging," *International Journal of Molecular Sciences* 22 no. 8 (April 2021): 3974.

10. S. F. Wu et al., "Role of Anxiety and Anger in Acne Patients: A Relationship with the Severity of the Disorder," *Journal of the American Academy of Dermatology* 18 no. 2 part 1 (February 1988): 325–33.

11. D. A. Rapp et al., "Anger and Acne: Implications for Quality of Life, Patient Satisfaction and Clinical Care," *British Journal of Dermatology* 151 no. 1 (July 2004): 183–89.

12. A. Rokowska-Waluch et al., "Stressful Events and Serum Concentration of Substance P in Acne Patients," *Annals of Dermatology* 28 no. 4 (August 2016): 464–69.

13. E. J. van Zuuren et al., "Rosacea: New Concepts in Classification and Treatment," *American Journal of Clinical Dermatology* 22 no. 4 (July 2021): 457–65.

14. H. Baldwin et al., "Evidence of Barrier Deficiency in Rosacea and the Importance of Integrating OTC Skincare Products into Treatment Regimens," *Journal of Drugs in Dermatology* 20 no. 4 (April 2021): 384–92; B. Medgyesi et al., "Rosacea Is Characterized by a Profoundly Diminished Skin Barrier," *Journal of Investigative Dermatology* 140 no. 10 (October 2020): 1938–50.e5.

15. M. Steinhoff, J. Schauber, and J. J. Leyden, "New Insights into Rosacea Pathophysiology: A Review of Recent Findings," *Journal of the American Academy of Dermatology* 69 no. 1 (December 2013): S15–26.

Chapter 12.
Five Elements Nutrition for Skin Beauty

1. Stephen L. DeFelice, "The Nutraceutical Revolution: Its Impact on Food Industry R&D," *Trends Food Science Technology* 6 (1995): 59–61.

2. P. Rajendran et. al., "Polyphenols as Potent Epigenetics Agents for Cancer." *International Journal of Molecular Science* 23 no. 19 (October 2022): 11712; S. L. Martin, T. M. Hardy, and T. O. Tollefsbol. "Medicinal Chemistry of the Epigenetic Diet and Caloric Restriction." *Current Medicinal Chemistry* 20 no. 32 (2013): 4050–59; M. Mirabelli et. al. "Mediterranean Diet Nutrients to Turn the Tide against Insulin Resistance and Related Diseases." *Nutrients* 12 no. 4 (April 2020): 1066; M. E. Obrenovich et. al. "Antioxidants in Health, Disease and Aging." *CNS and Neurological Disorders—Drug Targets.* 10 no. 2 (March 2011): 192–207.

3. A. Charlot et al., "Beneficial Effects of Early Time-Restricted Feeding on Metabolic Diseases: Importance of Aligning Food Habits with the Circadian Clock," *Nutrients* 13 no. 5 (April 2021): 1405.

4. M. Michalak et al., "Bioactive Compounds for Skin Health: A Review," *Nutrients* 13 no. 1 (January 2021): 203.

5. E. S. M. Abdel-Aal et al., "Dietary Sources of Lutein and Zeaxanthin Carotenoids and Their Role in Eye Health," *Nutrients* 5 no. 4 (April 2013): 1169–85.

6. A. P. Simopoulos, "The Importance of the Ratio of Omega-6/Omega-3 Essential Fatty Acids," *Biomedicine and Pharmacotherapy* 56 no. 8 (October 2002): 365–79.

7. J. T. Bamford et al., "Oral Evening Primrose Oil and Borage Oil for Eczema," *Cochrane Database of Systematic Reviews* no. 4 (April 2013): CD004416.

8. M. L. Dreher, and A. J. Davenport, "Hass Avocado Composition and Potential Health Effects," *Critical Reviews in Food Science and Nutrition* 53 no. 7 (2013): 738–50.

9. T. K. Lin, L. Zhong, and J. L. Santiago, "Anti-Inflammatory and Skin Barrier Repair Effects of Topical Application of Some Plant Oils," *International Journal of Molecular Science* 19 no. 1 (December 2017): 70; R. Chianese et al., "Impact of Dietary Fats on Brain Functions," *Current Neuropharmacology* 16 no. 7 (2018): 1059–85.

10. Y. Yoshioka et al., "Anti-cancer Effects of Dietary Polyphenols via ROS-Mediated Pathway with Their Modulation of MicroRNAs," *Molecules* 27 no. 12 (June 2022): 3816; J. Solway et al., "Diet and Dermatology: The Role of a Whole-food, Plant-based Diet in Preventing and Reversing Skin Aging—A Review," *Journal of Clinical and Aesthetic Dermatology* 13 no. 5 (May 2020): 38–43.

11. L. Pickart, J. M. Vasquez-Soltero, and A. Margolina, "GHK Peptide as a Natural Modulator of Multiple Cellular Pathways in Skin Regeneration," *Biomed Research International* (2015): 648108.

12. A. R. Vaughn et al., "Micronutrients in Atopic Dermatitis: A Systematic Review," *Journal of Alternative and Complementary Medicine* 25 no. 6 (June 2019): 567–77.

13. M. R. Mahmud et al., "Impact of Gut Microbiome on Skin Health: Gut-Skin Axis Observed through the Lenses of Therapeutics and Skin Diseases," *Gut Microbes* 14 no. 1 (Jan–Dec 2022): 2096995.

Chapter 13.
Chi Kung for Beautiful Hair

1. M. Grymowicz et al., "Hormonal Effects on Hair Follicles," *International Journal of Molecular Science* 21 no. 15 (July 2020): 5342.

2. K. D. Kaufman, "Androgens and Alopecia," *Molecular and Cell Endocrinology* 198 no 1–2 (December 2002): 89–95.

3. E. Kamp et al., "Menopause, Skin and Common Dermatoses. Part 1: Hair Disorders," *Clinical and Experimental Dermatology* 47 no. 12 (December 2022): 2110–16.

4. A. Rebora. "Telogen Effluvium: A Comprehensive Review." *Clinical Cosmetic and Investigational Dermatology* 12 (August 2019): 583–90.

5. Y. Bian et al., "Global Downregulation of Pigmentation-Associated Genes in Human Premature Hair Graying," *Experimental and Therapeutic Medicine* 18 no. 2 (August 2019): 1155–63.

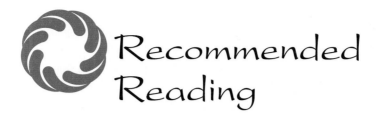 Recommended Reading

OTHER BOOKS BY MANTAK CHIA

Awaken Healing Energy through the Tao: The Taoist Secret of Circulating Internal Power. Aurora Press, 1991.

Cosmic Healing I: Cosmic Chi Kung. Universal Healing Tao Publications, 2001.

Healing Light of the Tao: Foundational Practices to Awaken Chi Energy. Rochester, Vt.: Destiny Books, 2008.

Healing Love through the Tao: Cultivating Female Sexual Energy. Rochester, Vt.: Destiny Books, 2005.

Iron Shirt Chi Kung. Rochester, Vt.: Destiny Books, 2006.

The Six Healing Sounds Taoist Techniques for Balancing Chi. Rochester, Vt.: Destiny Books, 2009.

Chia, Mantak and Kris Deva North. *Taoist Shaman Practices from the Wheel of Life.* Rochester, Vt.: Destiny Books, 2011.

——— and Christine Harkness-Giles. *Taoist Secrets of Eating for Balance: Your Personal Program for Five-Element Nutrition.* Rochester, Vt.: Destiny Books, 2019.

——— and Aisha Sieburth. *Life Pulse Massage Taoist Techniques for Enhanced Circulation and Detoxification.* Rochester, Vt.: Destiny Books, 2015.

——— and William U. Wei. *Cosmic Nutrition: The Taoist Approach to Health and Longevity.* Rochester, Vt.: Destiny Books, 2012.

INFORMATION ABOUT SKIN CARE

Draelos, Zoe, and Peter T. Pugliese. *Physiology of the Skin*, 3rd ed. Carol Stream, Ill.: Allured Publishing, 2011.

Hawkins, David R. *Power Versus Force: The Hidden Determinants of Human Behavior*. Carlsbad, Ca.: Hay House, 2002.

Schueller, Randy, and Perry Romanowski. *Beginning Cosmetic Chemistry: Practical Knowledge for the Cosmetic Industry*. Carol Stream, Ill.: Allured Publishing, 2009.

OTHER BOOKS BY ANNA MARGOLINA

Margolina, Anna, and Elena Hernandez. [New Cosmetology: The Foundational Principles of Modern Cosmetology]. In Russian. Moscow: Cosmetics and Medicine Publishing, 2012.

——— and Elena Hernandez. [New Cosmetology: Cosmetic Products]. In Russian. Moscow: Cosmetics and Medicine Publishing, 2015.

——— Elena Hernandez, and Anna Petrukhina. [Lipid Barrier and Cosmetics]. In Russian. Moscow: Cosmetics and Medicine Publishing, 2003.

Pickart, Loren, Anna Margolina, and Idelle Musiek. *Reverse Skin Aging: What Copper Peptides Can Do for You*. Cape San Juan Press/Summit Associates International, 2015.

About the Authors

MASTER MANTAK CHIA

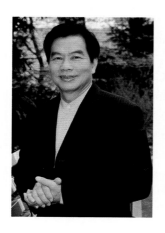

Mantak Chia has been studying the Taoist approach to life since childhood. His mastery of this ancient knowledge, enhanced by his study of other disciplines, has resulted in the development of the Universal Healing Tao system, which is now taught throughout the world.

Mantak Chia was born in Thailand to Chinese parents in 1944. When he was six years old, he learned from Buddhist monks how to sit and "still the mind." While in grammar school he learned traditional Thai boxing, and he soon went on to acquire considerable skill in aikido, yoga, and Tai Chi. His studies of the Taoist way of life began in earnest when he was a student in Hong Kong, ultimately leading to his mastery of a wide variety of esoteric disciplines, thanks to the guidance of several masters, including Master Yi Eng (I Yun), Master Meugi, Master Cheng Yao-Lun, and Master Pan Yu. To better understand the mechanisms behind healing energy, he also studied Western anatomy and medical sciences.

Master Chia has taught his system of healing and energizing practices to tens of thousands of students and trained more than three thousand instructors and practitioners throughout the world.

Stemming from his teaching corps, there are established centers for Taoist study and training in many countries around the globe. Master Mantak Chia has been the only person named twice by the International Congress of Chinese Medicine and Qi Gong (Chi Kung) as Qi Gong Master of the Year (in 1990 and 2012). He was also listed as number 18 of the 100 most spiritually influential people in *The Watkins Review* in 2012.

ANNA MARGOLINA, PH.D.

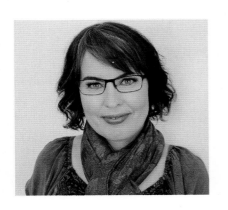

Anna Margolina, Ph.D., is a scientist and spiritual teacher as well as a Chi Kung and Universal Healing Tao instructor, speaker, and author. She has a degree in medical biophysics from the Russian Medical University and a Ph.D. in biology. Anna became interested in skin beauty in 1996 when she accepted a position as science writer and editor with the *Cosmetics and Medicine Journal* in Russia. Anna's job was to research the latest scientific information in the field of skin care and cosmetic products development. This work put her in touch with researchers and cosmetic manufacturers all around the globe and allowed her to develop a deep understanding of skin biology and functions.

In 2000 she published her first book, *The New Cosmetology,* which advocated for holistic and science-based skin care. Her following books were on cell therapies in skin care, hair care, and body shaping, as well as using healing oils for maintaining healthy skin (all published in Russia). She was a featured presenter at a number of international conferences and published dozens of articles in Russian. In 2001, Anna moved to the United States and started working as an independent scientific adviser for cosmetic companies in the United States and Israel. She has published newsletters, consulted with numerous women on scientifically based skin care, and presented at international skin-care conferences in Israel.

Anna became deeply interested in the magic of the mind-body connection, and in 2015 she started studying the practices of the Universal Healing Tao and traveled to Thailand to learn from Master Mantak Chia. In 2019, Anna became a Universal Healing Tao and Chi Kung certified instructor. Anna teaches Universal Healing Tao Chi Kung in Seattle, Washington.

The Universal Healing Tao System and Training Center

THE UNIVERSAL HEALING TAO SYSTEM

The ultimate goal of Taoist practice is to transcend physical boundaries through the development of the soul and the spirit within the human being. That is also the guiding principle behind the Universal Healing Tao, a practical system of self-development that enables individuals to complete the harmonious evolution of their physical, mental, and spiritual bodies. Through a series of ancient Chinese meditative and internal energy exercises, the practitioner learns to increase physical energy, release tension, improve health, practice self-defense, and gain the ability to heal him- or herself and others. In the process of creating a solid foundation of health and well-being in the physical body, the practitioner also creates the basis for developing his or her spiritual potential by learning to tap into the natural energies of the sun, moon, earth, stars, and other environmental forces.

The Universal Healing Tao practices are derived from ancient techniques rooted in the processes of nature. They have been gathered and integrated into a coherent, accessible system for well-being that works directly with the life force, or chi, that flows through the meridian system of the body.

Master Chia has spent years developing and perfecting techniques for teaching these traditional practices to students around the world through ongoing classes, workshops, private instruction, and healing sessions, as well as through books and videos and audio products. Further information can be obtained at universal-tao.com.

THE UNIVERSAL HEALING TAO TRAINING CENTER

The Tao Garden Resort and Training Center in northern Thailand is the home of Master Chia and serves as the worldwide headquarters for Universal Healing Tao activities. This integrated wellness, holistic health, and training center is situated on eighty acres surrounded by the beautiful Himalayan foothills, near the historic walled city of Chiang Mai. The serene setting includes flower and herb gardens ideal for meditation, open-air pavilions for practicing Chi Kung, and a health and fitness spa.

The center offers classes year-round, as well as summer and winter retreats. It can accommodate two hundred students, and group leasing can be arranged. For information on courses, books, products, and other resources, see below.

Universal Healing Tao Center
274 Moo 7, Luang Nua, Doi Saket, Chiang Mai, 50220 Thailand
Tel: (66)(53) 921-200
E-mail: universaltao@universal-tao.com
Website: universal-tao.com
For information on retreats and the health spa, contact:
Tao Garden Health Spa & Resort
Email: retreatreservation@tao-garden.com
Website: tao-garden.com

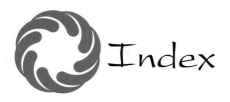

Index

Page numbers in *italics* refer to illustrations.